Sheila

To Sheila Jones and her family

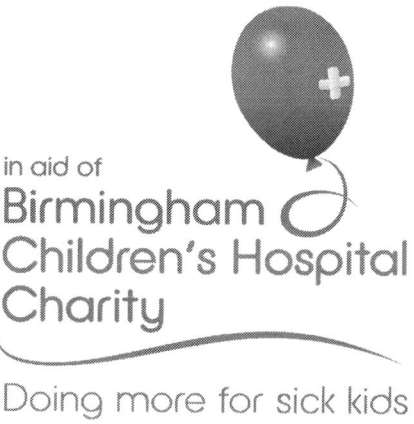

All royalties from the sale of this book go to the Birmingham Children's Hospital Charity.

Sheila
Unlocking the treatment for PKU

Anne Green

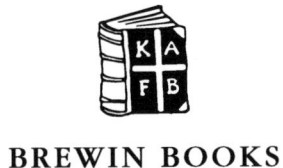

BREWIN BOOKS

BREWIN BOOKS
19 Enfield Ind. Estate,
Redditch,
Worcestershire,
B97 6BY
www.brewinbooks.com

Published by Brewin Books 2020

© Birmingham Women's and Children's Hospital Charity 2020

The author has asserted her rights in accordance with the
Copyright, Designs and Patents Act 1988 to be
identified as the author of this work.

Many of the historical photographs and documents used in
the preparation of this book are from the Hospital Archives and
are the property of Birmingham Children's Hospital. The holders
of copyright on uncredited figures are welcome to contact the
author or publisher who will make corrections in future editions.

All rights reserved. No part of this publication may be
reproduced, stored in a retrieval system, or transmitted in any
form or by any means, electronic, mechanical, photocopying,
recording or otherwise, without the prior permission in writing
of the publisher and the copyright owners, or as expressly
permitted by law, or under terms agreed with the appropriate
reprographics rights organization. Enquiries concerning
reproduction outside the terms stated here should be sent to the
publishers at the UK address printed on this page.

A CIP catalogue record for this book is
available from the British Library.

ISBN: 978-1-85858-714-1

Printed and bound in Great Britain
by 4edge Ltd.

CONTENTS

	Foreword	xi
	Abbreviations	xiii
	Acknowledgments	xiv
	Introduction	xvi
	Map of Birmingham	xviii
1.	THE FAMILY STORY – PART I: THE EARLY YEARS	1
	Mary	1
	Sheila 1949-1951	8
2.	BIRMINGHAM CHILDREN'S HOSPITAL	11
	The Early Years at Ladywood	11
	Profile: Leonard Gregory Parsons 1879-1950	12
	BCH 1951	13
	Profiles: Evelyn Marion Hickmans 1882-1972	14
	John Watson Gerrard 1916-2013	15
	Horst Bickel 1918-2000	17
	Sheila – Referral to BCH	18
3.	PHENYLKETONURIA	20
	Discovery of Phenylketonuria	20
	Early History of Phenylketonuria	22
4.	SHEILA – DIAGNOSIS	24
	The Ferric Chloride Test	24
	First Hospital Admission	25
	Specimen Collection	26
5.	THE BIOCHEMISTRY LABORATORY	28
	General Laboratory and Staffing	28
	Amino Acid Chromatography	30
	Dr Bickel's PhD	33

6.	**SHEILA – CONFIRMATION OF THE DIAGNOSIS**	35
	PKU Confirmed	35
	Mary's Persistence	35
7.	**SHEILA'S TREATMENT 1951-1953**	39
	Diet Preparation	39
	Second Admission to BCH	42
	Phenylalanine Free Diet	42
	Phenylalanine Reduced Diet	43
	Low Phenylalanine Diet at Home	44
	Phenylalanine Challenge	49
	Third Admission to BCH – Challenge Repeated	51
	1953 – What Next?	54
8.	**SHEILA 1953-1956**	55
	Further Cases at Birmingham	55
	Developmental Assessments	56
	Deteriorating Dietary Control	58
9.	**THE FAMILY STORY – PART II: THE 'LOST YEARS' 1956-1959**	61
	Life at Victoria Road, Aston	61
	Mary at Highcroft Hospital	64
10.	**SHEILA AT CHELMSLEY HOSPITAL**	66
	Context and History of Chelmsley Hospital	66
	Admission 1959	68
	The Early Years at Chelmsley	70
	Visit Home 1963	71
	Sheila and Mary	73
	Sheila after her Mum	75
	Sheila 1987	79
	Brooklands	81
	Reflections from the Staff at Chelmsley/Brooklands	83
	Sheila – A Tribute	83

11.	PKU DEVELOPMENTS	86
	Developments of Commercial Protein Substitutes	86
	Further Development of Diets and Paediatric Dietetics	88
	Demonstrating the Effects of Dietary Treatment	89
	Development of Newborn Screening for PKU: 1960-1970s	91
	Laboratory Assessment of Dietary and Biochemical Control	95
12.	RECOGNITION OF THE BIRMINGHAM CONTRIBUTION TO PKU TREATMENT	97
	The John Scott Award	97
	Who was John Scott?	97
	The John Scott Award 1962	98
	The 25th Anniversary Meeting of the John Scott Award – 1987	103
	The Sheila Jones Award 2018	104
13.	REFLECTIONS 2019	106
	Phenylketonuria Today	106
	Sheila's Life – from her Brothers	111
14.	CONCLUDING COMMENTS	118
	AFTERWORD	122
	APPENDICES	
I.	History of Birmingham	123
II.	History of Birmingham Hospitals	125
III.	Learning Disability Services in the UK	127
IV.	Extracts from Personal Notes	131
V.	The John Scott Award – Documents and Letters	136
	Personal Reflections by the Author	153
	Bibliography and References	156
	Index	166

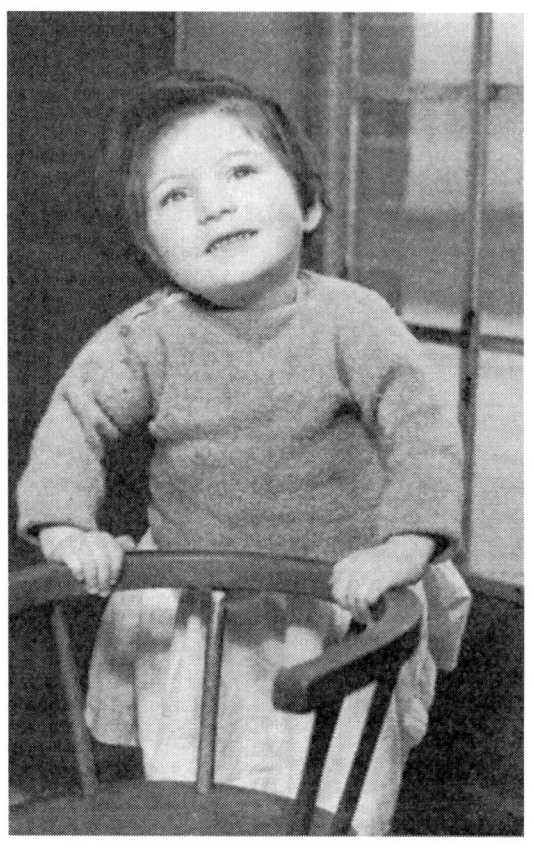

Sheila Jones was born in 1949 in Birmingham, UK. In 1951 she was referred to Birmingham Children's Hospital by the family doctor because of her slow development. She was diagnosed with Phenylketonuria (PKU) and was the first person to be given a diet to treat her condition. This is Sheila's story told with information from her clinical records, other original documents and the memories and help of Sheila's four brothers. It is a remarkable story and led to newborn screening for PKU in many countries, commercial production of special dietary products and treatment for those with PKU across the world. Sheila's contribution to the now successful treatment for those with PKU is immense. Sadly, Sheila herself did not benefit long term and died at the age of 49 years in Birmingham. This is her story.

Mary Jones (1951)
*'It's not fancy investigations I want,
when are you going to treat my child?'*

* * *

Dr Horst Bickel (1951)
*'The mother's perseverance gave me no chance
to rest on the strength of a fine diagnosis.'*

* * *

Professor John Gerrard (1987)
*'If only we had known we were helping her
more than we understood at the time.'*

* * *

Dr Brian Oliver (1987)
Consultant Psychiatrist, Chelmsley Hospital
'We will have to ensure that she is publicly acknowledged.'

AUTHOR BIOGRAPHY

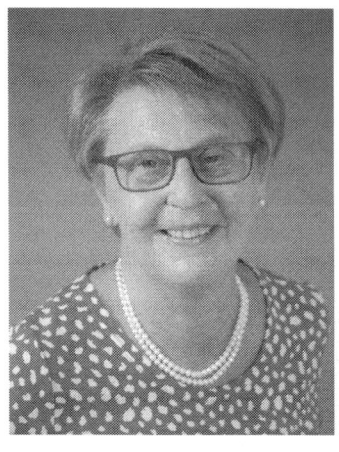

Anne Green BSc, MSc, PhD, FRCPath, FRCPCH, FRSC, FRSB had a distinguished career as a Paediatric Clinical Biochemist in the UK National Health Service based at Sheffield Children's and Birmingham Children's Hospitals. She was Head of Department of Paediatric Biochemistry/Consultant Clinical Chemist (1982-2006) at Birmingham Children's Hospital (BCH) with responsibility for the Newborn Screening Programme and Inherited Metabolic Disorders Services for the West Midlands region, and succeeded Dr Noel Raine (1963-1980), Harold Salt (1953-1961) and the first Biochemist Dr Evelyn Hickmans (1923-1953). She has made major scientific contributions and published widely in the fields of Newborn Screening and Inherited Metabolic Disorders, including Phenylketonuria (PKU), and became Professor of Paediatric Biochemistry at the University of Birmingham in 1994. She lectured and taught at numerous international conferences, was secretary of the Society for the Study of Inborn Errors of Metabolism and co-founder of both the British Inherited Metabolic Disorders Group and the National Metabolic Biochemistry Network (MetBio.Net). She held the post of Lead Scientist for the UK National Newborn Screening Centre from 2006 until 2011.

FOREWORD

I am delighted to contribute a few words for this fascinating and moving story of Sheila Jones and her family. The discoveries made at the Birmingham Children's Hospital in the early 1950s have a unique place in the history of Phenylketonuria (PKU). The demonstration of the successful dietary treatment of this otherwise devastating inborn metabolic disorder still stands as an exemplar of a disorder which if detected early can be effectively treated by 'correcting' the metabolic abnormality. The dietary treatment of PKU also provided the momentum for the establishment and development of newborn screening programmes across the world. For these reasons alone, the importance of the work done in Birmingham in the 1950s cannot be overemphasized.

I too was born in 1949 in Birmingham, in Dudley Road. I remember the Kings Norton and Harborne of those days, from going to birthday parties of a school friend, along with many other places mentioned in Sheila's story. I remember too how my family was proud of how Birmingham's National Health Service grew and, of course we all went to the Birmingham Children's Hospital with our problems.

While the scientific achievement of Drs Bickel, Gerrard and Hickmans is well recognised, the story of Sheila herself and her family is less well known. We are fortunate that in Dr Anne Green we have an author who has had an outstanding career as a biochemist in providing newborn screening as well as diagnosing and treating patients with metabolic diseases at Birmingham Children's Hospital. Throughout her career she met and got to know many of those directly involved in the story: Dr Bickel, Dr Gerrard and members of their laboratory team, medical and nursing staff who looked after Sheila, and Sheila herself. With unique contributions from Sheila's family and historical documents she has produced a book which not only weaves together the background history of the hospital, the scientific work of the three medical and scientific pioneers, but also the story of Sheila. We learn about what happened to her, her family, and the challenges they faced and the sacrifices they made during the socially deprived and uncertain times through which they lived. This book movingly tells the story of a family and their contribution to the history of PKU.

It provides not only a very readable and well written account of the science but also has dealt sensitively with the issues which the family endured. It reminds us of the huge developments which have followed over the 70 year lifetime of the NHS.

Those with PKU and their families will immediately understand its importance to their lives but it should also be read by all health professionals working in newborn screening, inherited metabolic disorders, genetics and beyond. Every disease has a series of chapters in its history – this is a chapter of PKU which resulted in the transformation of a condition that caused profound brain damage resulting in severe learning difficulties to a chronic disease which can be effectively managed. This unique account from Birmingham Children's Hospital adds immeasurably to that history.

Professor Dame Sally Davies
Master of Trinity College Cambridge
Former Chief Medical Officer of England

March 2020

ABBREVIATIONS

ACB	Association of Clinical Biochemists / Association for Clinical Biochemistry and Laboratory Medicine
BCH	Birmingham Children's Hospital
DHSS	Department of Health and Social Security
DQ	Development Quotient
E.S.PKU	European Society for Phenylketonuria and Allied Disorders
FSU	Family Services Unit
GB	Great Britain
GI	Gastrointestinal
GRO	Government Records Office
ICI	Imperial Chemical Industries
IQ	Intelligence Quotient
IMD	Inherited Metabolic Disorders
ISNS	International Society for Neonatal Screening
LIU	Light Industrial Unit
MRC	Medical Research Council
NHS	National Health Service
NSPKU	National Society for PKU
AH	Phenylalanine Hydroxylase
PAL	Phenylalanine Ammonium Lyase
PHE	Public Health England
PKU	Phenylketonuria
PPA	Phenyl Pyruvic Acid
RAMC	Royal Army Medical Corps
SSIEM	Society for the Study of Inborn Errors of Metabolism
WRVS	Women's Royal Voluntary Service
WWI	World War I
WWII	World War II

ACKNOWLEDGMENTS

This book would not have been possible without help from many people. Firstly thank you to several individuals at BCH, in particular Dr Fiona Reynolds, Chief Medical Officer; Mary Anne Preece, Consultant Paediatric Biochemist/Director of Newborn Screening; the Clinical Chemistry Department staff (past and present); Professor Anita McDonald, Consultant Paediatric Dietitian; Ann Daly, Library Manager and Natalie Powell, Video Services Manager. Thanks also to staff at Brooklands Hospital, in particular Dr Ashok Roy, Consultant Psychiatrist and Margaret Matthews, Unit Manager. I am grateful to the Birmingham Women's and Children's Hospital Charity for funding this publication and a special thank you to Dame Sally Davies and Sir Muir Gray for their words.

I would like to thank the colleagues and families of John Gerrard in Canada and Horst Bickel in Germany for help checking details and provision of photographs and additional information.

My husband Richard encouraged me to write this story and gave me so much help and advice. Most importantly he chivvied me along to keep focussed, thus enabling me to complete a task dear to my heart which had lingered for far too long. I thank him for his unstinting support and patience.

Most of all thank you to Sheila's brothers, Terry, Trevor, Philip and Liam for their extreme generosity and willingness to share their memories, family information and feelings, which have enabled me to make this a very special story. In the summer/autumn of 2016 we met to piece together Mary's and Sheila's lives for us all to appreciate. A special thank you goes to Trevor and Marylyn (Mel), for welcoming me so warmly to their home; on my numerous visits we sat and chatted about Sheila, her mother Mary, and their life in Birmingham over cups of coffee and delicious cake. The added dimension of the family story in Birmingham, as the context for the scientific events described by Drs Gerrard, Hickmans and Bickel enables a greater appreciation of the pioneering work which took place.

Thanks also to Tom Day, Consultant Biochemist (retired) for recounting real stories about what actually happened almost 70 years ago and to Christine Clothier, Paediatric Dietitian (retired) for filling in historical details about the early diets. Professor Carl Chinn's help on the history of Birmingham and permission to use photographs from his archive are very much appreciated. I would also like to pay tribute to 'others' who in some way have contributed to

Sheila's story but for whom it has not been possible to record their respective contributions: the laboratory staff who worked with Evelyn Hickmans and those who assisted Horst Bickel – Brian Rudd and Anne Whitehouse.

I have very much appreciated the help and expertise of Alistair Brewin at Brewin Books and his understanding and patience in bringing this book to production.

Thank you Terry, Trevor, Philip and Liam for your welcome and friendship and for sharing your family story with me and allowing me to write this book. It has been a privilege.

INTRODUCTION

If you have Phenylketonuria (PKU), have a family member with PKU, are a health professional working in the area or simply just curious you might have wondered how did the dietary treatment for PKU come about. How did newborn screening become established? This is the story about where it all started with a little girl Sheila, born in 1949, who had PKU.

Sheila was diagnosed in 1951 at the age of two years by doctors at Birmingham Children's Hospital (BCH) where they developed a special dietary treatment for her PKU. The findings of this first treatment are documented scientifically in several publications, however little has been known about Sheila's early life and family background in Birmingham. Since 1956, following the dietary trial, she has been 'lost in the system' and her whereabouts, and what had happened to her have remained unknown. Who was Sheila and what happened to her family?

In 1987, a chance discovery came about when testing blood and urine by the Clinical Chemistry Department at BCH from a 37 year old female inpatient at a local mental institution, Chelmsley Hospital. These tests revealed she had the disorder Phenylketonuria and it was subsequently confirmed that this lady, Sheila Jones, had been the very first patient in the world to be treated with a diet in the early 1950s at BCH. Following this discovery I met Sheila in 1987 and followed her care over the ensuing years until her death 12 years later in 1999, when I was honoured to deliver a tribute at her funeral. I later got to know Sheila's brothers Terry, Trevor, Philip and Liam. Sadly, Sheila's mother Mary had died in 1981. I have interviewed and chatted with Sheila's brothers and with their kind permission, understanding and unstinting help I have put the medical/scientific story about Sheila's life in Birmingham into a family perspective. Interest from health professionals and families with PKU, who wanted to know more about Sheila, encouraged me to write this story and share previously untold information in order to appreciate the circumstances and context of Sheila's life.

Background and reference material are largely UK based to reflect the local context for the story, and a map of Birmingham in 1959 is included with relevant locations numbered. Specific references and more general reading are grouped together into sections, according to subject matter, within a combined listing at the end of the book. Where information from a specific reference has been included in the text, the author and year of publication is listed in brackets with reference details included in the combined listing.

As well as published material I have been privileged to have access to historical documents, personal notes, photographs and clinical records about Sheila from BCH and Chelmsley Hospital. Original unpublished historical documents and records of personal communications, audio recordings, photographs and videos which have been used in writing this story will be archived in Birmingham Central Library for future reference and safe keeping as part of the BCH Archive. Clinical records remain in the keeping of BCH. Permissions to reproduce photographs and illustrations are acknowledged individually, all others being part of the BCH Archive.

In part I have used Sheila's brothers' own words and tried to create a picture of their family life. I have also had numerous discussions with various health professionals from Chelmsley Hospital who remember Sheila and others who were working there at that time. Words spoken, or written, by others and reproduced in the story are written in *italics*. Throughout Sheila's story the medical language in use at that time is used.

This is a remarkable story of a brave little girl and a courageous, determined mother coupled with the pain, hardship, sadness and family sacrifice they experienced. It provides an historical and family based story of the impact of this important scientific innovation. I have included other related events, including the subsequent international recognition of this pioneering treatment. I have reflected on the major developments for PKU which have followed as a result of Sheila's treatment in the 1950s, as a reminder of what has been achieved over the last 70 years.

The story is told chronologically and had she lived, Sheila would have been 70 years old when this text was completed in 2019.

Sheila must not be forgotten as we reap the rewards of her legacy.

Professor Anne Green

December 2019

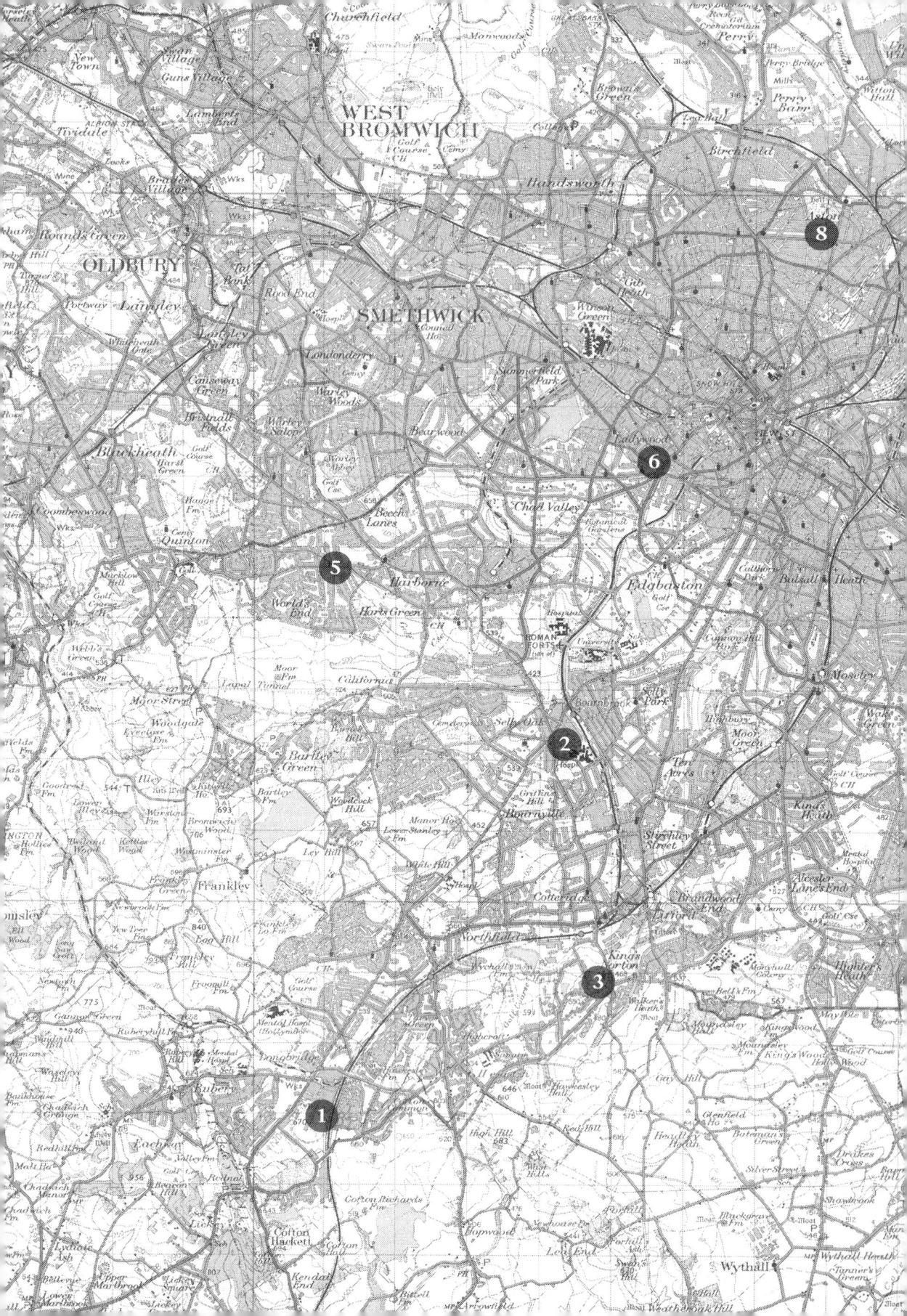

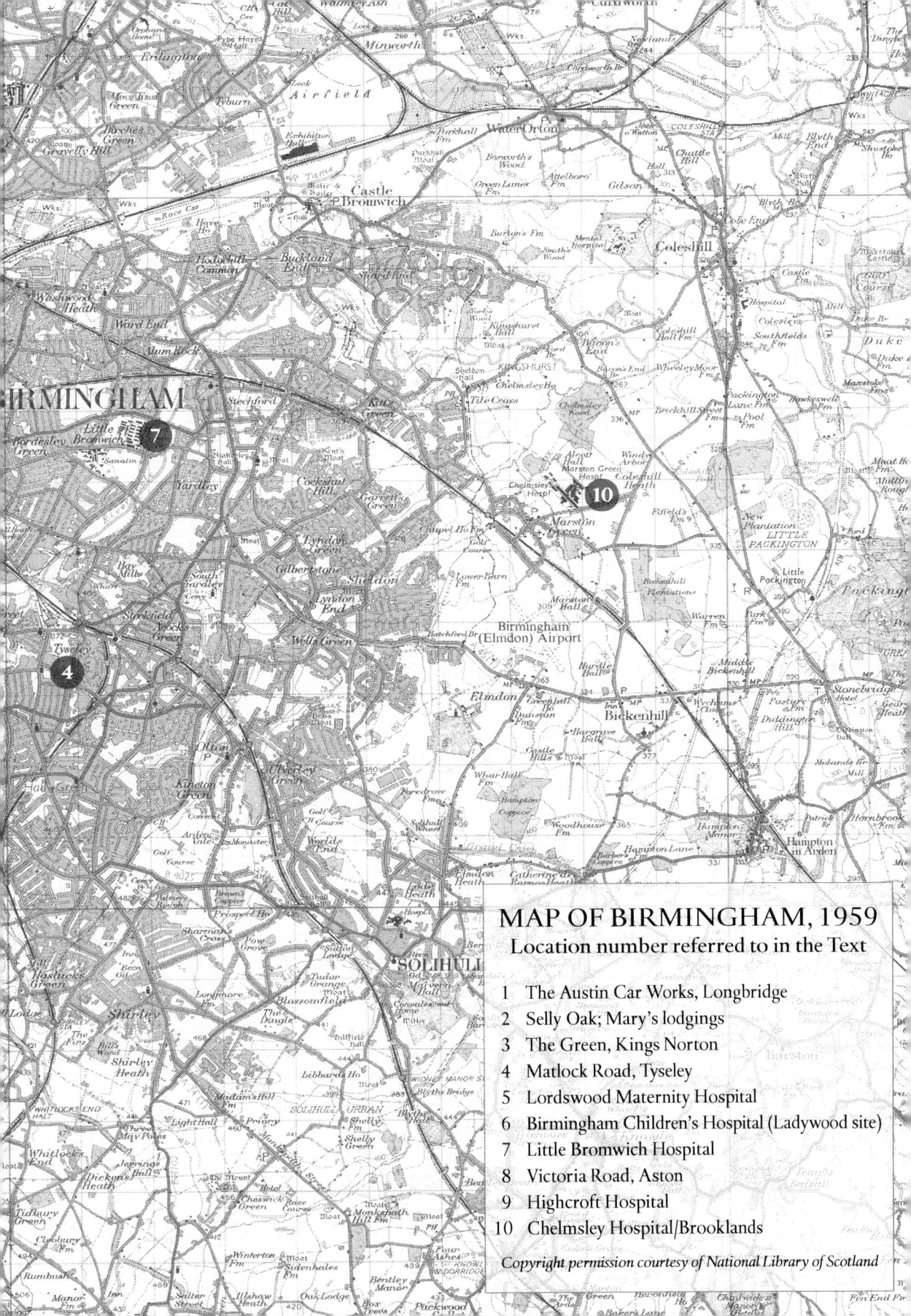

Trevor Jones – Sheila's Brother (2018)
*'Our Mum had it hard without help from anyone.
She kept the family together.'*

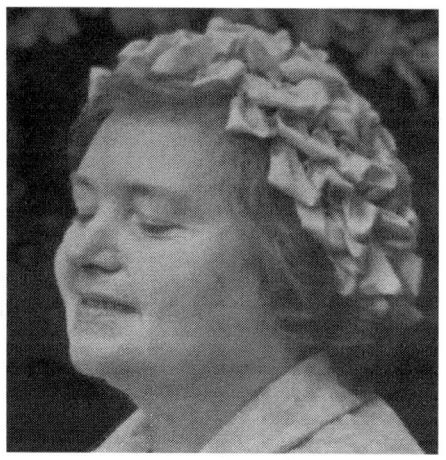

Mary Jones 1971
1st January 1917 – 8th October 1981

(Photograph kindly provided by the Jones Family)

1

THE FAMILY STORY – PART I: THE EARLY YEARS

Terry and Trevor Jones: *'She was never a normal little girl'*.

Mary
The family story begins in Ireland with the birth of Sheila's mother, Mary. Mary Margaret (Philomena) Rooney was born in Magheramore, Kinlough in County Leitrim in the north-west of Ireland on 1st January 1917. Mary was brought up in the Catholic faith and Philomena was her communion name. In the early 20th century Ireland was a poor country with the majority of people living in the countryside, in small country towns and villages. Levels of poverty were exceptionally high especially in the rural communities. In the early 1920s there was often no running water, no electricity and poor sanitation. Mary was from a large farming family who lived at Pollboy (An Poll Buí), a townland to the west of Manor Hamilton, County Leitrim, and was the eldest of six children; her father was Patrick Rooney and mother Katie McCue. Mary would have gone to a local school and after leaving school and being the eldest it would have been especially important for her to find employment to help the family. The economic climate in the country was poor, with few industries and spiralling unemployment, making it virtually impossible to find paid work in the rural areas where most women worked on the family farm. Mary initially left home around 16 years of age to go to Dublin and had found work possibly in a hotel or 'in service' with a family.

Because of these difficulties during the 1930s and 1940s the rate of emigration from Ireland, especially for single women, was high in the quest to find work. The advent of World War II (WWII) in 1939 had resulted in Britain desperately needing labour to help the war effort and the government organised large scale recruitment of workers. At the outbreak of WWII Birmingham was a large highly industrialised city of 1 million people (see Appendix I) and its huge industrial output became focussed on the war effort, and firms such as ICI (Imperial Chemical Industries) and the Austin Motor Company sent recruiting agents to Ireland. The majority of Irish migrants recruited in the 1940s were young single women like Mary. She came to Birmingham around 1942/3 to work at the car works (fondly known in Birmingham as *'The Austin'* works) located in Longbridge, south Birmingham (see Map Birmingham, 1). The exact circumstances, other than the need for employment, which brought about her move are not fully known as she never went back to visit Ireland and there was no subsequent contact with her family in Manor Hamilton.

When Mary arrived in Birmingham the Longbridge site had been converted from a car manufacturers into an aircraft factory for the war effort, and this is where Mary had obtained a job as a drilling machinist.

Birmingham was an obvious target for enemy action. More than 2,000 people were killed and swathes of the city were destroyed in aerial bombing raids. For Mary, arriving in a country at war, in a city which was being heavily bombed, this must have been a very threatening environment for a young single girl on her own. She initially lived in lodgings in Selly Oak (see Map Birmingham, 2) a suburb in

The Austin Motor Works c.1930. The site showing the outside of the factory (photograph courtesy of Birmingham Libraries).

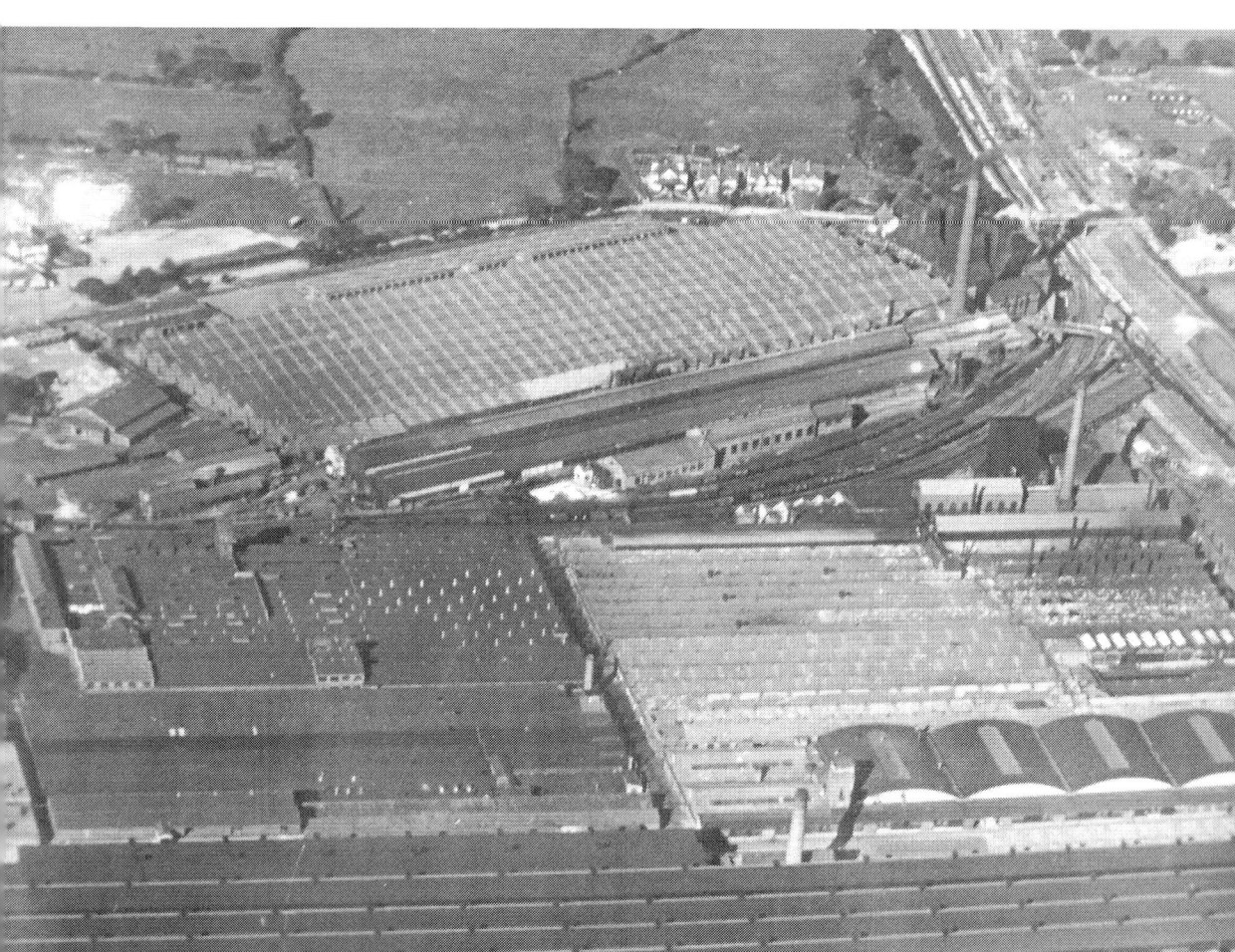

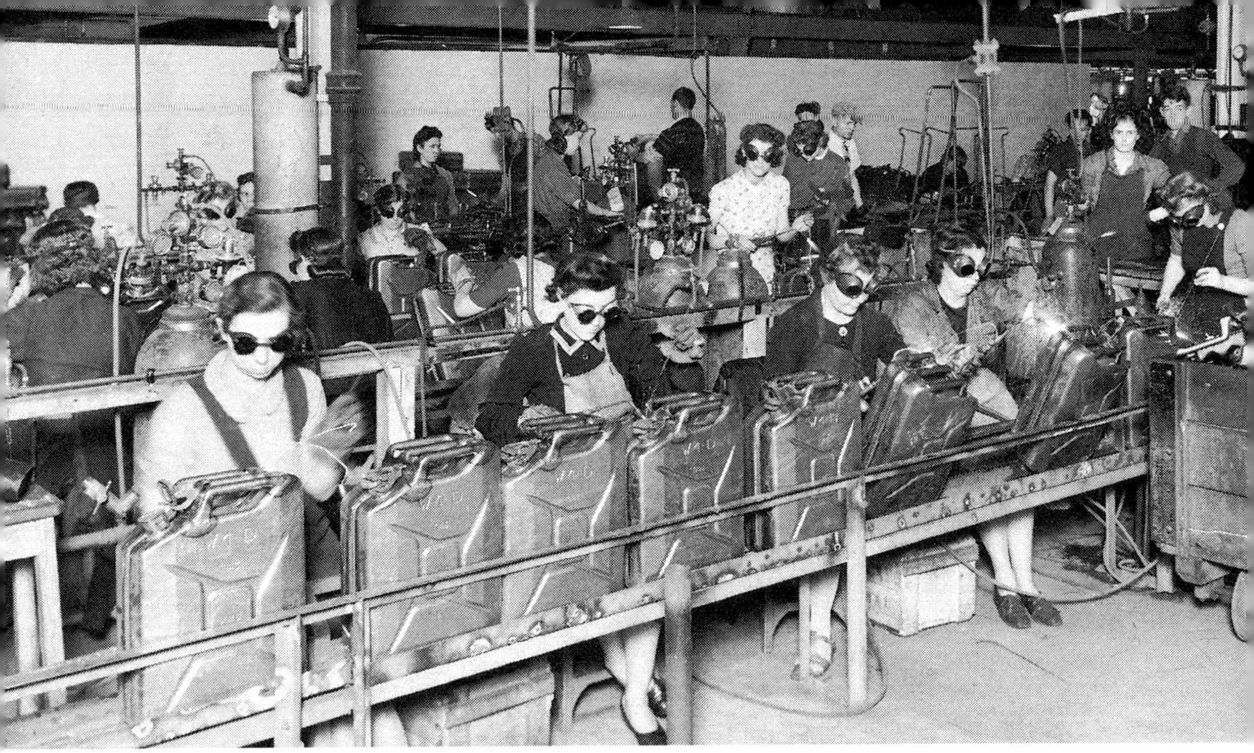

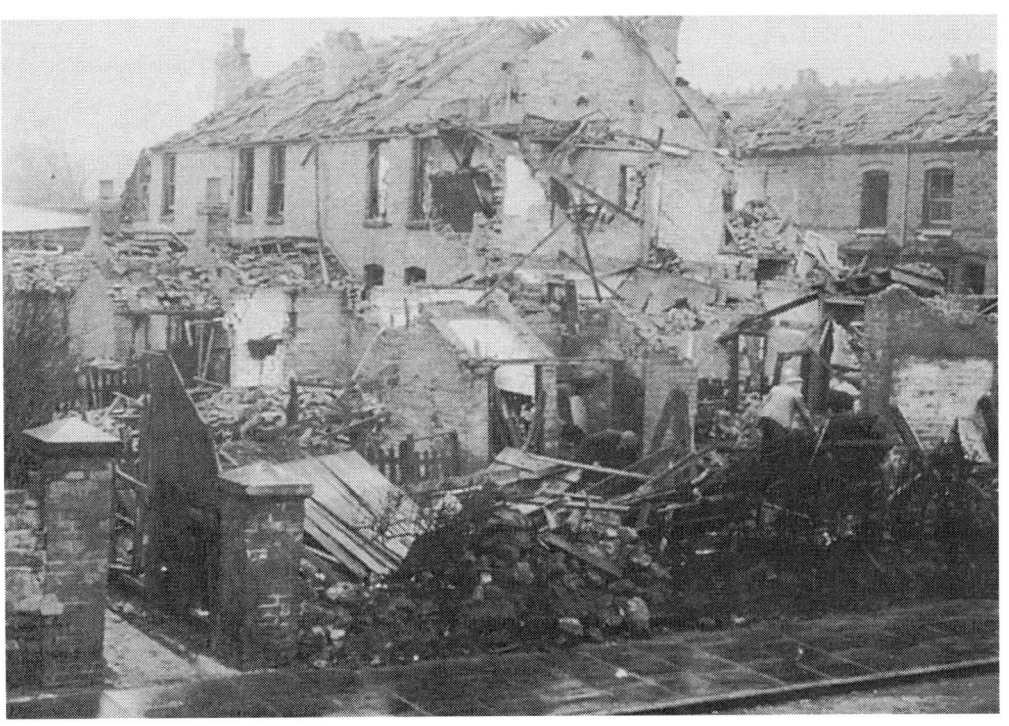

Women workers on an assembly line at Austin works, 1943 (photograph courtesy of Alton Douglas).

Bomb damage in Selly Oak (photograph courtesy of Alton Douglas).

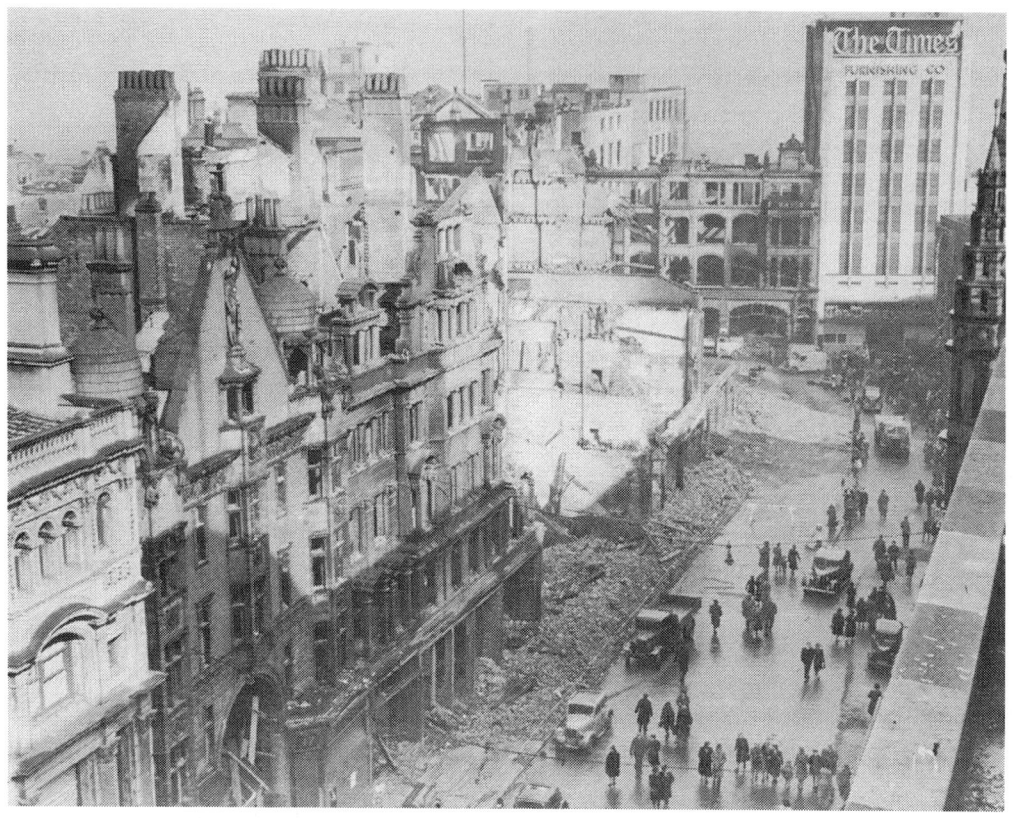

Birmingham: devastated inner city (photograph courtesy of Alton Douglas).

south Birmingham just a few miles from Longbridge. The blackouts and bombing raids would have been an enormous contrast to the rural family life where she had been brought up. At war's end Birmingham was left with a devastated inner city in which housing was poor and scarce and, like many other cities in Europe, with few resources to rebuild.

After the war ended in May 1945, Mary married Edgar James Jones at St Edwards Church, Raddlebarn Road, Selly Park, Birmingham and lived around the village green (89, The Green) in the nearby area of Kings Norton (see Map Birmingham, 3). They had a son, Terry who had been born in 1945 at the hospital at Dudley Road (see Appendix II). Kings Norton was a pleasant 'village' with a parish church, picturesque cottages, a pub, a cinema and several shops; number 89 was one of a row of small cottages on a road running up towards the church, called 'the Twatlins' – a derivation of Watling Street (Caswell 1997; Pearson 2004) – with a general store at the end of the row and the church at the top.

1. The Family Story – Part I

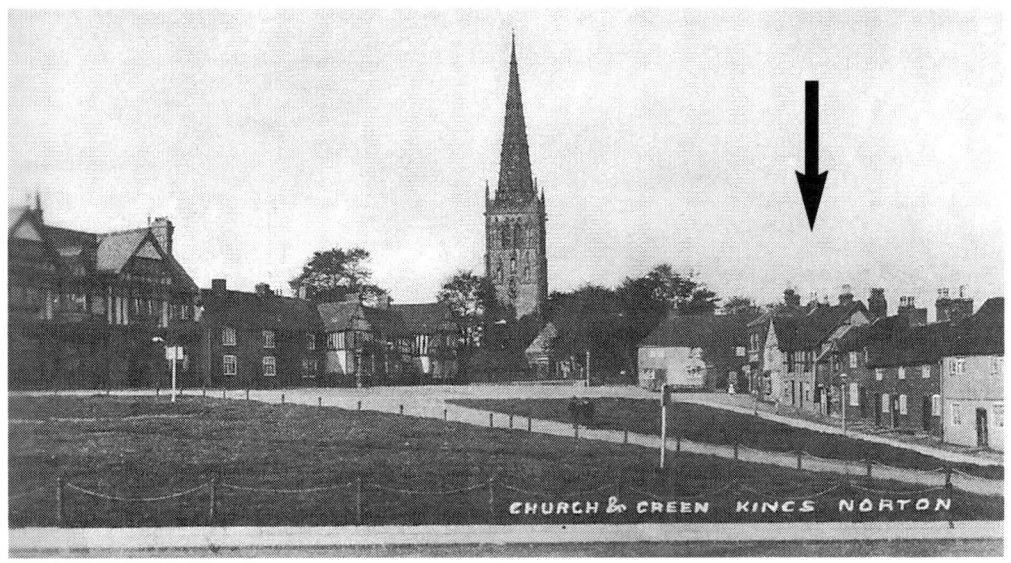

The Green, Kings Norton c.1920 with number 89 highlighted (photograph courtesy of Birmingham Libraries).

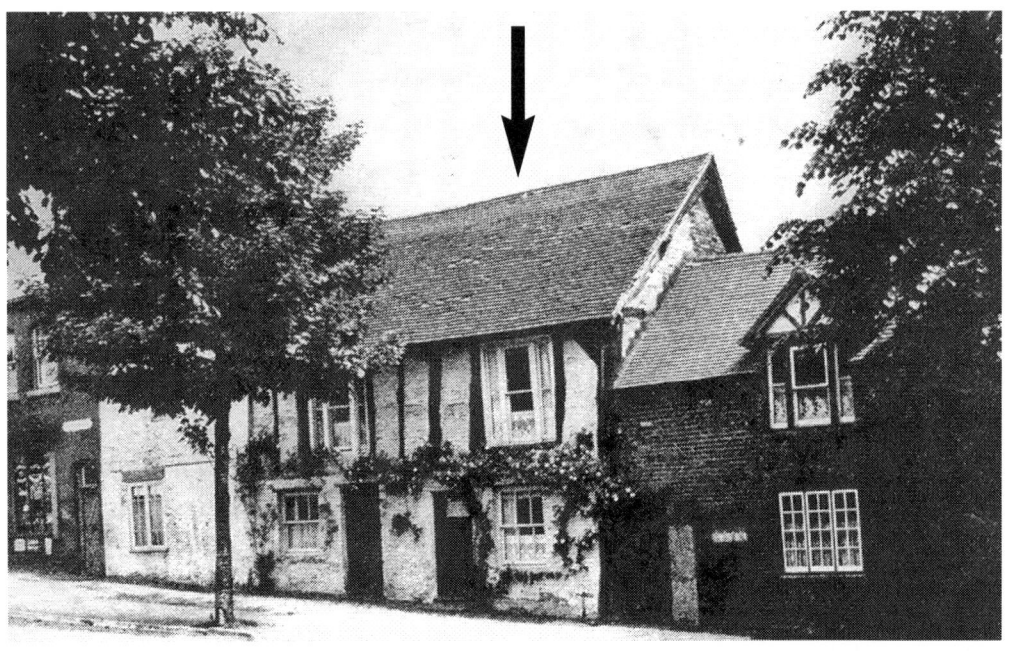

Kings Norton Cottages c.1935 including 89 (photograph courtesy of Birmingham Libraries).

The cottages were subsequently demolished in the 1950s/early 1960s. In 2019 the 'gap' where the car park entrance is now located is the site of the former cottage, number 89. It was facing The Green and close by the Church. Terry can remember the cottage and in particular sitting outside eating a piece of cake whilst people walked past on their way to Church and proudly saying *'my Mum made this'*.

Sadly the Jones' marriage broke down and Mary became a single mother. She continued to live at The Green and her second son Trevor was subsequently born in 1948 at Highcroft Hospital, Erdington (see p.64), which, at that time soon after the end of the war, was being used as a Maternity Hospital.

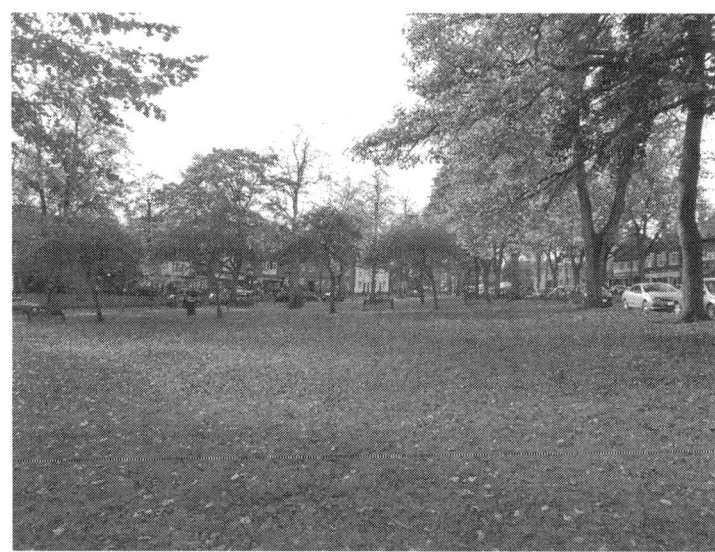

Right: View of The Green 2019, from former site of no 89.

Below: Former site of number 89, The Green, Kings Norton 2019.

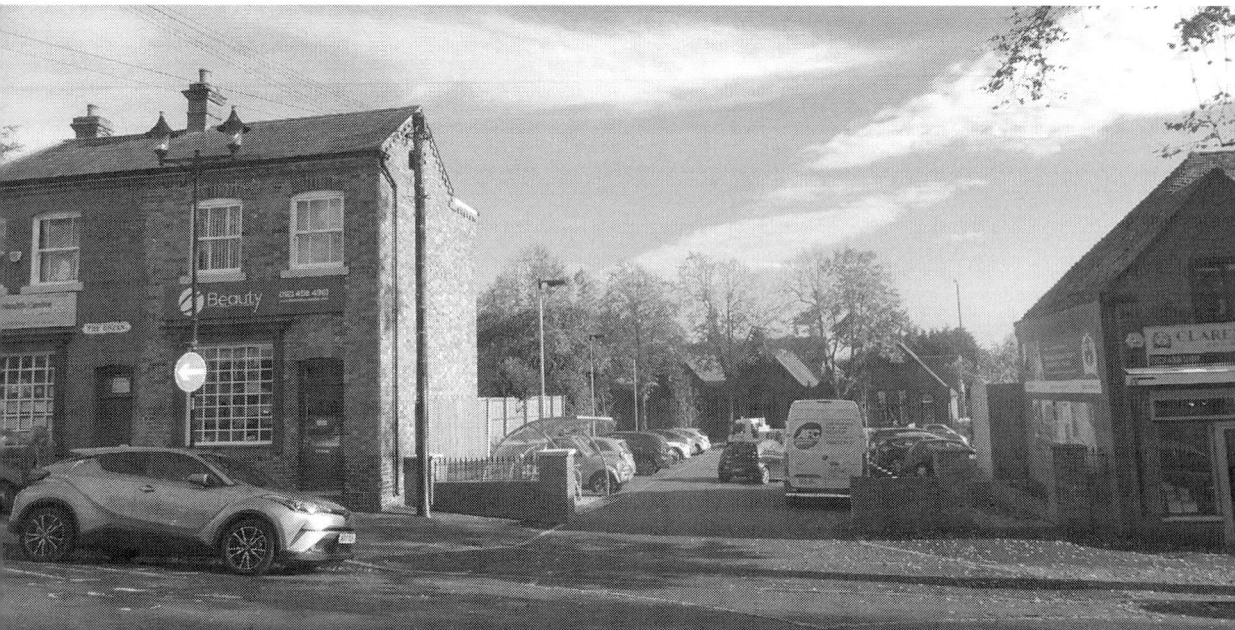

1. The Family Story – Part I

Around 1948/1949 Mary and her two sons, Terry and Trevor, moved to Matlock Road, Tyseley in south-east Birmingham about six miles from the city centre (see Map Birmingham, 4). This is a long crescent shaped road and at the bottom there is a block of maisonettes where the family lived in a modest ground floor flat. The same house is still there in 2019. In post war Birmingham many families in the city were living in poverty and food rationing continued until 1954. In contrast to many other inner city areas, however, Matlock Road was a relatively pleasant environment and the maisonette had a small kitchen, living room, two bedrooms, inside toilet and bathroom with hot and cold water. Considering there was such poverty and housing shortage in the city Mary was better placed than

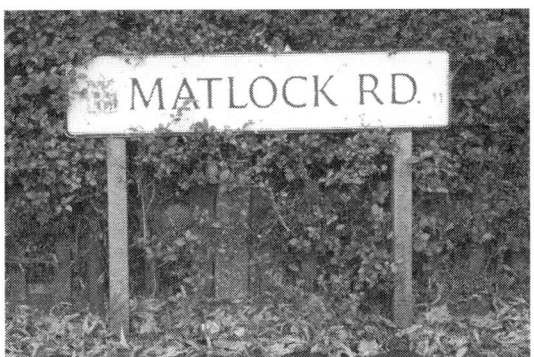

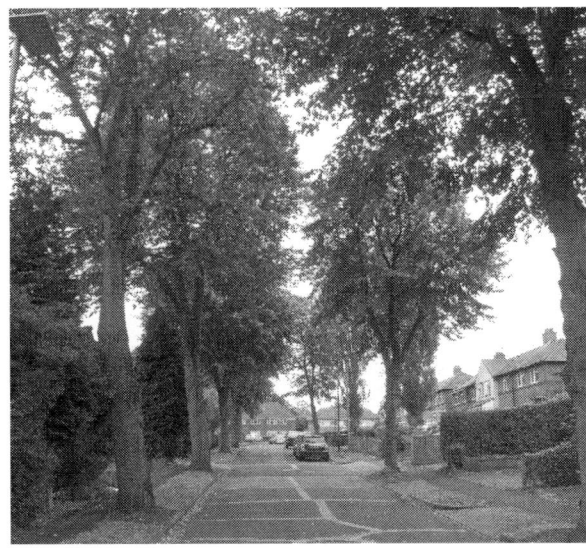

Above & Right: Matlock Road, Tyseley, 2019.

Below & Below Right: 33/3 Matlock Road, Tyseley, 2019.

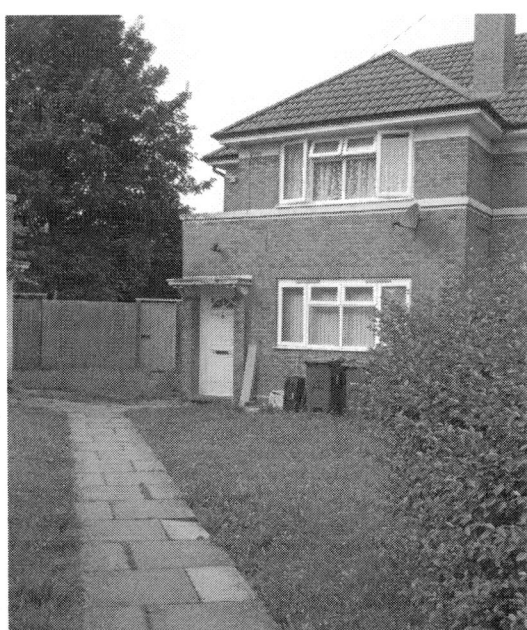

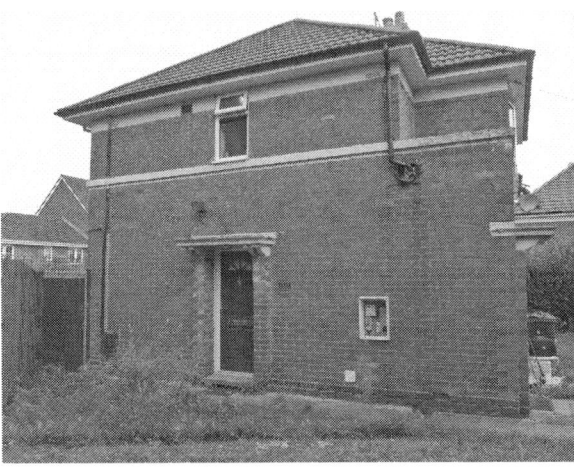

many others at that time. Terry and Trevor speak with affection about their home at Matlock Road and remember walking down the footpath to the side door of their ground floor flat and playing on the grassy area in front of the two storey block. This was the world into which Sheila Jones was born.

Sheila 1949-1951
Sheila was born on 2nd October 1949 at 44 Lordswood Road (Lordswood Maternity Hospital) in Harborne, Birmingham. Lordswood Maternity Hospital started life as a private house built in 1856 and subsequently became a Voluntary Hospital (May 1915) during World War I; this convalescent hospital treated over 2000 casualties. In 1928 it became Lordswood Residential Nursery for the care of 30-40 children under the age of two years. At the outbreak of WWII the nursery was evacuated and from the mid-1940s was used as a maternity hospital until its closure in 1968. It has since been demolished but is roughly on the same site as the current Lordswood Medical Practice (see Map Birmingham, 5).

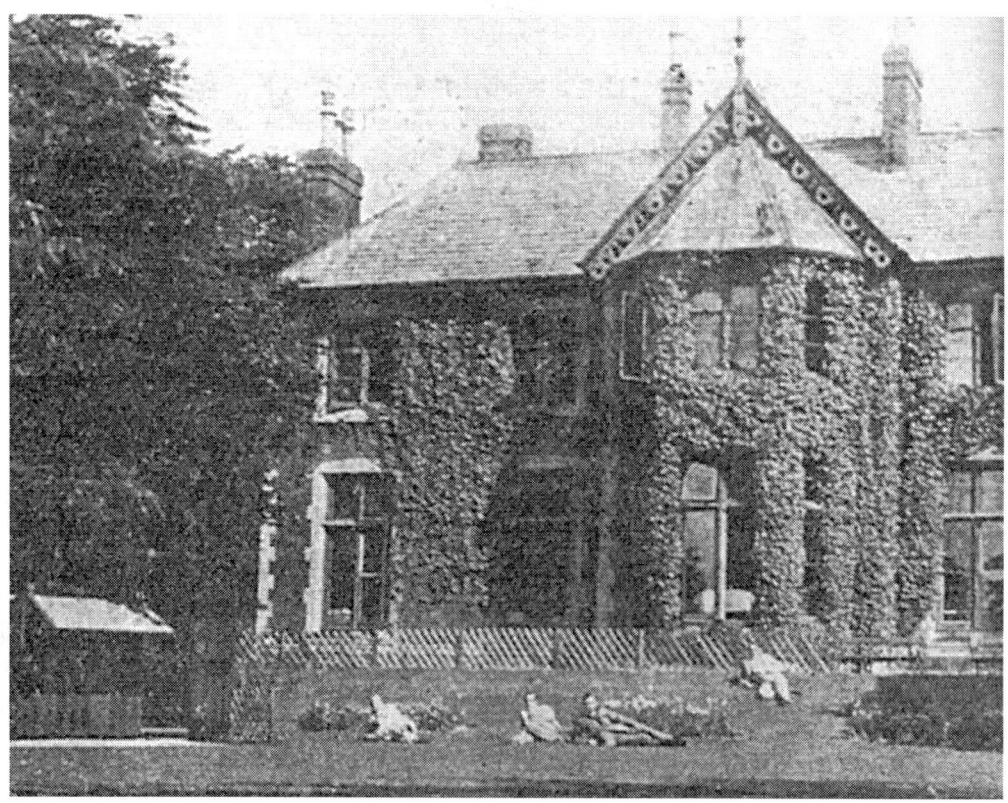

Lordswood Maternity Hospital (photograph courtesy of Harborne Society).

1. The Family Story – Part I

It is unclear why Mary gave birth at this hospital, as Lordswood Road is some distance and at the opposite side of the city from her home at Matlock Road, except that post war there was a shortage of maternity places. Both of Sheila's older brothers had been born in different hospitals across the city. We do not know much information about Sheila's birth other than she was born normal at term, with a birth weight of 3.7kg; her birth certificate states her mother as Mary Jones with no father named. There is no mention of any pre-natal or immediate post-natal medical problems in subsequent clinical records and it appears that Sheila came home after a few days to Matlock Road to live with her mother and her two brothers, Terry now aged four years and Trevor only one year old. Mary was delighted that she now had a lovely daughter.

Mary had had no contact with her parents and family since she had left Ireland. She had no family support in Birmingham to help with her young family; the children had no grandparents at hand, no aunts or uncles nearby and no father around. Mary no longer had her job at the car works, and although they had a nice maisonette, the family were poor with little or no income to support the family. Trevor recalls *'we had very little and our clothes were like a bag of rags'*.

For a brief period, there were two lodgers at Matlock Road, presumably as a source of income for the family but also because of the extreme housing shortage post war, when it was common for lodgers to have the 'spare' room. Sheila's brothers recall that the lodgers had the best and larger bedroom at the back of the maisonette whilst their Mum had the smaller room with themselves in bunk beds and Sheila initially in a cot – *'it wouldn't surprise me if Mum slept on the settee at times'*. Later: *'Sheila must have slept with our Mum in the same bed'*. They have memories of Sheila sleeping with Mary, who was trying to comfort her daughter.

The brothers recall very little from Sheila's early months as they were very young with Trevor only a year older than Sheila. She was a strong and healthy, well nourished baby and all was well at first; a pretty little girl with blonde hair and brown eyes. However it soon became clear that all was not normal with her, and her brothers have memories of unusual features of her behaviour developing –*'she used to grab a blanket, sit on the floor on the blanket and rock to and fro'* – this rocking motion became a consistent feature. *'Sheila didn't like having clothes put on – just liked being on a blanket'*. From an early age she was very destructive and the brothers particularly remember coming into the kitchen in a morning where *'it was just a mess – with flour and tea on the kitchen floor. She used to pull things off shelves'*. The young boys were both at a local nursery at Reddings Lane and don't know what Sheila would do during the day; Sheila never went to nursery as Mary needed to be constantly watching over her. They recall that Sheila sometimes would really enjoy something you were doing – *'she would hit out and bang the floor with her hands wanting you to do it again and again – wanted you to do it more'* – it was an excitement for her which she communicated by making noises and movements but never words. Another thing they remember is that if Sheila hurt herself she didn't seem to feel pain.

In their words *'she was never a normal little girl'*, *'she never spoke'*; Trevor recalls: *'I used to say to Mum – do you think she will ever get better?'*

This was Mary's third child so she must have known Sheila was not developing as she should and she must have been very concerned about her daughter with the question in her mind *'was she normal?'* and worried that something was amiss. It was for this reason that she took Sheila to see the local family doctor, Dr Allin, in nearby Fox Hollies Road, when she was around one year old. The doctor recognised that Sheila's mental development was slow; she had not started to sit until about nine months and was backward in various other aspects of her development. Dr Allin referred Sheila to Birmingham Children's Hospital for an opinion.

2

BIRMINGHAM CHILDREN'S HOSPITAL

A new site was found in Ladywood Road only a little further out of town, off Broad Street, and with a large space at the back for future development. 'It was a beautiful site' said one enthusiastic speaker at the following Annual General Meeting; 'it faced the right way and was on a tram route' (Waterhouse 1962).

The Early Years at Ladywood
The 'new' Children's Hospital (see Appendix II) where Sheila was referred in 1951 had been opened in 1917 on the Ladywood site on the west side of the city (see Map Birmingham, 6) with the first patients arriving on Christmas Eve; events surrounding World War I had frustrated the building timetable so the hospital was only partially completed. In 1918, with the end of WWI, came huge developments made possible by medical staff returning from the war with new ideas of scientific medicine and increasing specialisation in consultant practice.

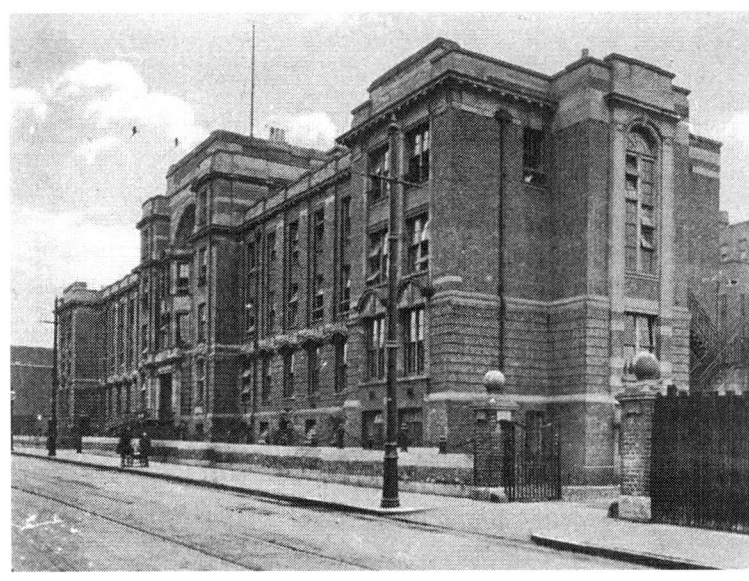

Birmingham Children's Hospital (Ladywood Site) c.1950s.

There were many major advances and achievements in clinical medicine during the ensuing years, particularly the changing landscape of infectious diseases brought about by the discovery and introduction of antibiotics. Immediately after WWI with only a few wards open there was about 100 beds but this had risen to 167 by 1928. Further expansion, with the building of an isolation block and a baby block, increased beds to around 300. The wards had been built facing south-east with large south facing windows and balconies overlooking lawns and gardens. A key figure during all of this development, and of particular relevance to this story, was one of the early medical pioneers at BCH during the Ladywood years, Leonard Parsons (see Profile).

Sir Leonard Gregory Parsons (1879-1950)

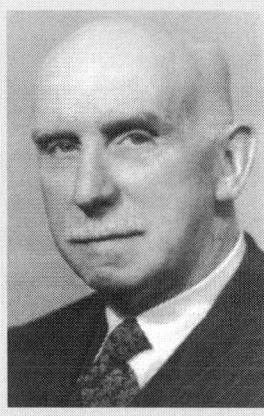

Leonard Parsons.

Leonard Parsons was born in Aston, Birmingham and educated at King Edward VI Grammar School, Birmingham and Mason College Birmingham University. In 1910 he was appointed to Birmingham Children's Hospital as Physician to outpatients and was subsequently appointed as lecturer in paediatrics at Birmingham University; in 1928 he became the first Professor of Child Health (1928-1946) at the University of Birmingham. He received a Knighthood in 1946 and was made a fellow of the Royal Society in 1948.

Leonard Parsons had recognised the importance of research using scientific investigations in the study of children's diseases of the day. Laboratory facilities had become a necessity and the Ladywood site allowed space for their development; until then the hospital had had to depend on the University laboratories. It was this approach and foresight which led to the establishment of chemical laboratory investigations at BCH, and the appointment of Evelyn Hickmans as the first biochemist for the hospital in 1923, and only the second biochemist to be employed in a hospital in England (Broughton and Lines 1996). Leonard Parsons' areas of interest were many but included nutritional disorders, especially rickets, scurvy and anaemias of childhood, and he was responsible for the high standards of research at that time. He harnessed the use of the new developments in pathology and biochemistry to benefit the study of children's disorders to great advantage.

2. Birmingham Children's Hospital (BCH)

When Leonard Parsons retired in 1946, James Maclure Smellie (1893-1961) was appointed. James Smellie was born on 19th May 1893, son of James Smellie of Pedmore, Worcestershire. He studied Medicine at Edinburgh and after a period in the Royal Army Medical Corps (RAMC) he held posts in Edinburgh and London. His special interests in children led to his appointment in 1922 as Physician to Outpatients at BCH. He served as a medical officer during WWII and returned to civil practice in 1946 when he was appointed to the first whole time post of Professor of Paediatrics and Child Health at Birmingham University, succeeding Sir Leonard Parsons when he retired.

Under the clinical leadership of Leonard Parsons and then James Smellie, BCH had become a specialist centre where new developments requiring laboratory testing could take place. It was to this hospital at Ladywood where Sheila was referred into a clinical environment which enabled the pioneering work which led to her treatment.

BCH 1951
By the late 1940s, after the end of the World War II, the hospital was expanding and had several new specialties. It had become part of the newly formed National Health Service (NHS) in 1948 and together with the General, Queen Elizabeth, Women's, Maternity, Nerve and Dental Hospitals became part of the United Birmingham Teaching Hospitals Group. With the change in organisation from essentially voluntary to being under the umbrella of a regional hospital board constitution, there were obvious changes. The hospital had become a teaching centre for undergraduate medical students and nurses with formal ties to the University. On the professional side there was a welcome and much needed growth in the number of consultant paediatric physicians and an active research environment. The close relationship and interdependence of the various branches of medicine characterised this post war period. This was the scene for three professionals who had each been attracted to work at BCH – one chemist and two physicians – and together they were the key to the subsequent development of Sheila's story.

Dr Evelyn Hickmans (see Profile) had expanded the original biochemistry department to a larger laboratory and provided the expertise for the subsequent laboratory work which was so critical for Sheila's diagnosis and treatment.

Dr John Gerrard (see Profile) a physician returned from World War II was a recently appointed Reader in Paediatrics (academic position at the University of Birmingham) with hospital consultant status. His chief was James Smellie, Professor of Paediatrics. As part of his duties, Dr Gerrard had developed a special outpatient clinic for children with mental retardation.

Dr Horst Bickel (see Profile) was a young doctor from Germany embarking on a PhD at the University of Birmingham, based at BCH, and who remarked on his arrival: *'I was surprised by the high standards of Paediatrics in this English hospital'* (Bickel 1996).

Evelyn Marion Hickmans (1882-1972)

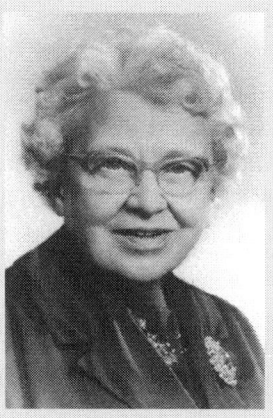

Evelyn Hickmans c.1962.

Evelyn Marion Hickmans was born on 9th April 1882 in Sedgefield near Wolverhampton, the daughter of a dairyman David Hickmans and his wife Mary. She had two sisters and a brother.

She gained a scholarship to Birmingham University where she was awarded a BSc in Chemistry in 1905 and an MSc a year later. She was one of the very few women at the time to study chemistry, and one of only 27 who attended Birmingham University between 1880 and 1949. She then went to London University to study household science and became interested in dietetics. In 1919 she went to Toronto University as a lecturer in applied chemistry and dietetics. She came back to Wolverhampton from Toronto in 1922 most likely because her mother was ill; her mother died that year.

Dr Leonard Parsons was Evelyn's cousin and he had asked her to join him to work at the Children's Hospital with the purpose of establishing chemical assays to support his work. Leonard Parsons was a keen researcher who had recognised the importance of laboratory tests. In 1923 Evelyn Hickmans established the first Paediatric Biochemistry Laboratory in the country when she was appointed to BCH. She made many original contributions and pioneered the development of Paediatric Biochemistry; she gained a second MSc in 1923, this time in biochemistry, and a PhD in physiology in 1925 both at Birmingham University. Her early work centred on developing assays to investigate patients of Dr Parsons with coeliac disease, and to understand the different kinds of rickets. She developed microanalysis techniques and was quick to develop new methods suitable for use with the small blood volumes obtained from young children. This partnership between chemist and physician reflected Leonard Parsons' interests in marasmus and childhood anaemias and resulted in highly productive research with many publications.

In the late 1940s she introduced paper chromatography (then in its infancy) for the study of amino acids. Her laboratory at BCH became one of the few places in the UK where this technique was being applied successfully in a hospital setting. A series of meetings were arranged so that other laboratory workers across the country could learn about the technique. It was this initiative that catalysed the setting up of a formal association for biochemists working in a hospital environment and at Birmingham Children's Hospital on 15th December 1949 the Midlands Association of Clinical Biochemists was inaugurated. Dr Hickmans' laboratory gained an international reputation. She retired in 1953 but continued to contribute to the teaching of laboratory science locally for many years.

Dr Hickmans was also a founder member of Wolverhampton Soroptimists Club and Wolverhampton branch of the Association of University Women. She never married and died unexpectedly on 16th January 1972.

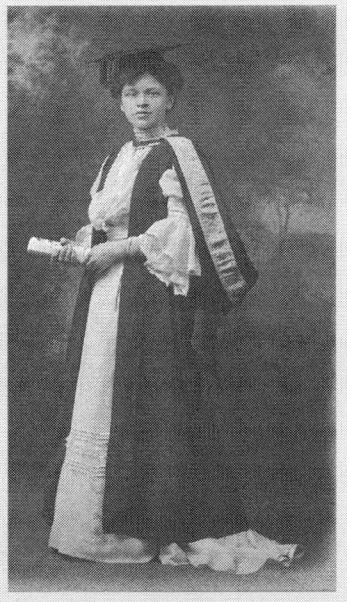
Evelyn Hickmans' Graduation.

John Watson Gerrard (1916-2013)

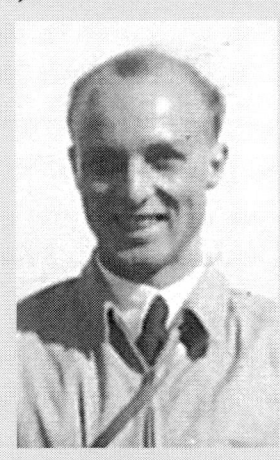
John Gerrard c.1950.

John Gerrard was born on 14th April 1916 in Northern Rhodesia (now Zambia) the son of Herbert Shaw Gerrard, a medical missionary and his wife Doris Gerrard (née Watson). He grew up in England and in 1941 graduated in medicine from Oxford. He then went to work in Birmingham where he met and got to know Dr Leonard Parsons and his son Clifford. He was there for a six months 'clerkship' before joining the British Army where he worked as a Medical Officer during World War II and served in North Africa, Italy and Palestine. After he was demobbed he was encouraged by Leonard Parsons to take up Paediatrics and returned to Birmingham to a training post at Birmingham

Children's Hospital in the mid/late 1940s with Professor Smellie. Dr Gerrard became a consultant at BCH in 1951.

One of his specific roles was to have an outpatient clinic for children with mental retardation. At that time the only preventable form of mental retardation known about was 'cretinism' (hypothyroidism) which could be treated with thyroid replacement therapy. There were also children with 'mongolism' (now known as Down's Syndrome or Trisomy 21) which was then recognised as a cause of mental retardation. There were also many other children for whom there was no diagnosis. Other forms of preventable or treatable mental retardation were not known at that time.

Dr Gerrard moved from Birmingham to Saskatchewan, Canada in the summer of 1955 having had a six months period in Johns Hopkins University, Baltimore. He became head of the Department of Paediatrics in Saskatoon serving in that capacity until 1971. He retired from the department in 1983. In 1985 he received the Alan Ross award from the Canadian Paediatric Society for his renowned contributions to child health care, education, research and advocacy. He was made an Officer of the Order of Canada in 1998, one of the country's highest honours. He died on 3rd March 2013.

The author gratefully acknowledges the help with these details from Jon Gerrard, Canada (photographs kindly provided by the Gerrard Family).

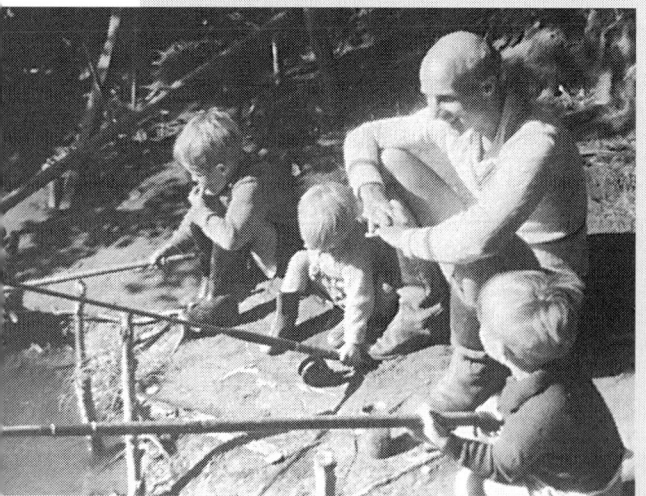

John Gerrard with sons Jon, Peter and Chris c.1954.

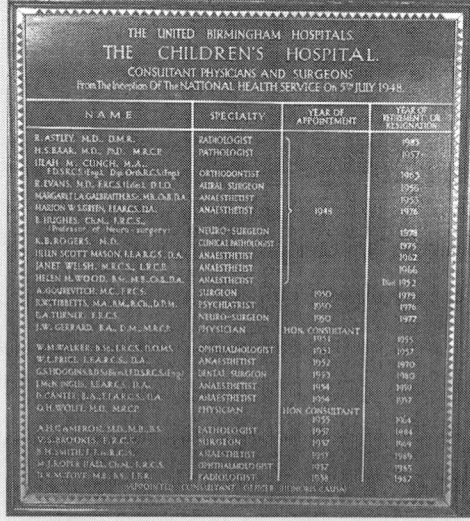

BCH Honour board 1948-1958.

Horst Bickel (1918-2000)

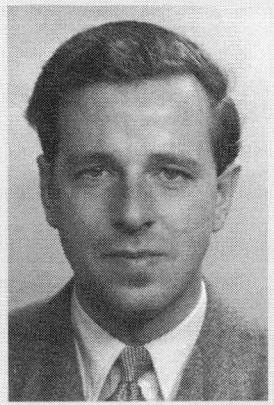

Horst Bickel c.1950.

Horst Bickel was born on 28th June 1918 in Hamburg and trained as a medical doctor in Berlin, Lausanne and Freiburg and then, after the start of World War II, went to Innsbruck and Vienna for his clinical studies where he qualified in 1942. From early 1943 he served in the German navy as a medical officer until the end of the war. During WWII he worked as a doctor in military hospitals and went to sea on a minesweeper, and at the end of the war a hospital ship*. Dr Bickel survived the war and resumed his medical training in 1945 at the Hamburg Children's Hospital on a voluntary basis. About a year later he developed tuberculosis and initially went to a sanatorium in Switzerland.

Just before the outbreak of WWII Horst had met his wife-to-be, Stella, a young student from Oxford, whilst holidaying on the Adriatic coast, when he had reputedly stole her deckchair! She was incensed with this ungentlemanly behaviour but he apologised so profusely that this was the beginning of their romance! They were able to meet a few times in Berlin and London before war broke out. He obviously made a lasting impression and when the war was over Stella joined the Red Cross in order to be able to go to Germany and search for him, and then followed him to Switzerland where she nursed him back to health in an alpine hut near Davos.

After recovering from his illness in 1947 he was unable to return to the hospital at Hamburg but was able to continue his Paediatric training with Professor Guido Fanconi at the University Children's Hospital Zurich, Switzerland. It was there that he became interested in aminoacidurias and chromatography and in order to gain more experience was drawn to Birmingham in 1949 to take up a research post. The study of aminoacidurias was an area of interest that had been developed at BCH by Professor Sir Leonard Parsons and Dr Evelyn Hickmans. This would have been a most unusual step for a German doctor to go to a post in England so soon after the war – but he was able to bring his wife Stella back to her homeland. They lived in Solihull just outside Birmingham.

From October 1949 to March 1952 Dr Bickel studied for his PhD at BCH under the supervision of Professor Smellie whilst in receipt of a Medical Research Council Grant. His research topic was the study of amino acid patterns in plasma and urine from normal children and those with various disorders; this was an important and new application of amino acid chromatography to clinical situations. His work was undertaken with the help of Evelyn Hickmans and her laboratory staff. Dr Bickel obtained his PhD from Birmingham University in 1952 with his thesis: *Aminoaciduria in Childhood*.

Dr Bickel left Birmingham in 1954 to continue his Paediatric career in Germany, initially in Marburg and then Heidelberg. He had a distinguished career both nationally and internationally in the field of inherited metabolic disorders continuing to study and develop services for PKU and newborn screening. In 1972 he became an honorary member of the British Paediatric Society and in 1983 an honorary member of the Royal College of Physicians. In 1988 he was awarded the Order of the Federal Republic of Germany. He died on 1st Dec 2000.

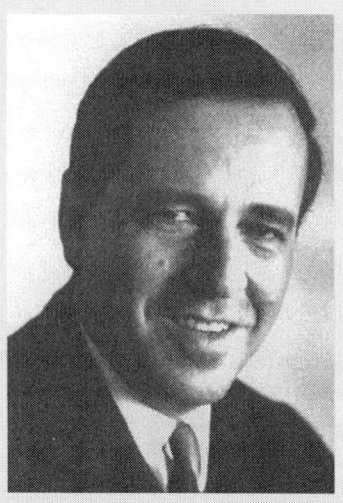

Horst Bickel c.1970s.

* *Horst Bickel was colour blind and therefore he was not forced to serve in a military capacity but was able to go to sea as a medical officer.*

The author gratefully acknowledges the help with these details from Susan Bickel, Germany; Michael Liberra, Germany; Professor Friedrich Trefz, Reutlingen; and Professor Georg Hoffmann, Heidelberg (photographs kindly provided by Susan Bickel, Germany and Georg Hoffmann, Heidelberg, Germany).

Sheila – Referral to BCH

Following the referral from her GP, Sheila was seen at BCH (she was now 17 months old) in the special outpatient clinic of Dr Gerrard's on 13th March 1951. Dr Bickel was also working as a young doctor in the clinic as part of his research.

The clinical details of Sheila's presentation to BCH, and her subsequent diagnosis and dietary trial, are published in the scientific literature and the details below and later in the book are taken directly from these publications. However, they are supplemented with information from personal notes and anecdotes from various professionals involved at the time (see Appendix IV) and Sheila's two older brothers Terry and Trevor.

2. Birmingham Children's Hospital (BCH)

At the time of her referral Sheila was badly brain damaged and could not stand or walk and had no speech. She had clearly been well looked after by her mother, Mary, and was well nourished and had no abnormal physical signs, apart from rough skin with some eczema on her face. She lay in her cot crying and groaning for hours at a time and rocked continuously rolling her head from side to side and banging it on the pillow. She had fair hair, and had an unusual 'mouse like' smell. The doctors thought these features were suggestive of Phenylketonuria (PKU), a relatively newly described disorder at that time, and so Mrs Jones was asked to bring a sample of Sheila's urine to the clinic. It was noted that Sheila had two older brothers who were both mentally normal. Mary reported that Sheila's father (who did not live with the family) was healthy and there was no consanguinity. Mary was asked to bring the urine specimen the following week but did not return and so a letter was sent to her at home with a container for the urine. She subsequently brought a sample of Sheila's urine to the out-patients department some weeks later, on 14th April (by coincidence John Gerrard's birthday!).

3

PHENYLKETONURIA

'The discovery raises two important questions: (1) whether some other types of mental illness will not be found to have hereditary biochemical backgrounds and (2) how far the course of such illnesses, when identified, can be influenced by the deliberate alteration of body metabolism' (Penrose 1946).

Discovery of Phenylketonuria
In 1951 although Phenylketonuria was a known cause of mental defectiveness it was a relatively new disorder whose history had begun in Norway in the 1930s. Its discovery had come about because of an encounter between a biochemist/physician and a distraught and tenacious mother. A story not dissimilar to this one.

In 1934 Dr Ivar Asbjørn Følling discovered what we now know as Phenylketonuria or PKU. Dr Følling had trained as a chemist and also as a physician at Oslo University and therefore understood that diseases could result from a failure of metabolism. He was asked to see a brother and sister aged four years and seven years. The two children both had severe mental retardation, a peculiar odour, eczema, restlessness and fair hair. Their unhappy mother had asked for help at many institutions but had got no explanation for her children's condition; she had noticed that the peculiar musty smell always clung to her children. Driven by the mother's persistence and determination she sought help from Dr Følling.

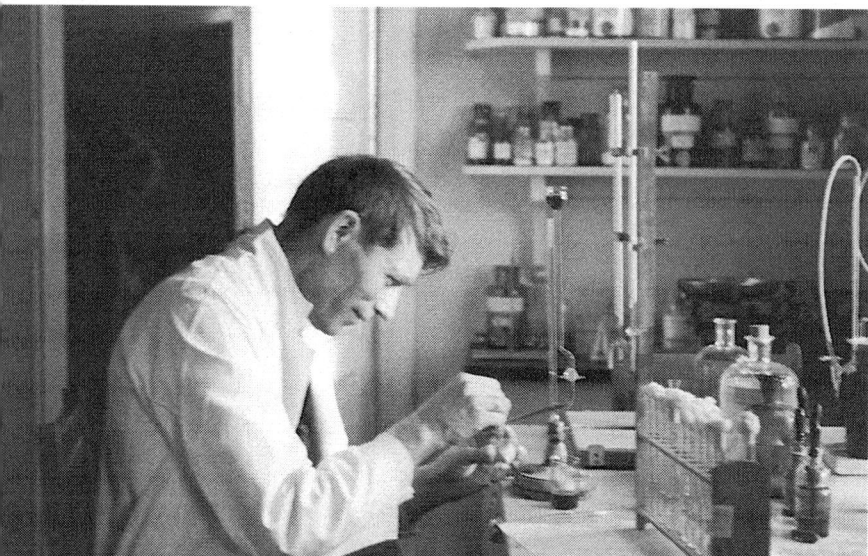

Dr Ivar Asbjørn Følling (1888-1973) c.1930s (photograph kindly provided by the Følling Family).

As part of his investigations Dr Følling used a chemical, ferric chloride, to test the urine from these two children. This was a simple test which was normally used to test for ketones in the urine in diabetes, and associated with a sweetish smell to the urine. This was not a test used at that time in patients with mental retardation and we can only assume it was performed because of the unusual smell in the two children – an inquisitive idea from a chemist. He added the ferric chloride to each urine and was surprised when both urines turned an olive-green colour which disappeared a few minutes later; normal urine stayed a yellowy/brown colour and Dr Følling had never seen this green colour before and it was not described in the literature. To check that it was not caused by any medications he withdrew medication from the children and repeated the testing a few days later; the urines still turned this unusual olive-green colour. This suggested to Dr Følling that there was an unknown substances in the urine. In order to find out what was causing this unusual colour he asked the mother to collect large quantities of urine from her two children. Several weeks later, using 20 litres of urine, he used chemical methods to isolate pure crystals which he showed, by study of their melting point, to be phenylpyruvic acid (PPA). A connection between the presence of PPA and the cause of the children's mental retardation was suggested.

Dr Følling was curious about whether there could be others with this same finding. He visited institutions for the mentally retarded, collected urine from 430 patients, and found eight more cases (with three instances of recurrence in siblings) with this 'green' ferric chloride reaction. He hypothesized that in these patients, who were all regarded as feebleminded, there was an excess amount of the amino acid phenylalanine in the body and this was converted to PPA and spilled over into the urine. He called this newly discovered condition *imbecillitas phenylpyruvica* and postulated that it was recessively inherited, in view of the association in siblings and consanguinity in four families.

Others were motivated to look for cases of this new disease and soon after Dr Følling's initial report George Jervis, an American physician and biochemist, described similar cases but used the term *phenylpyruvic oligophrenia*. Lionel Penrose, a Psychiatrist from Colchester, UK described more cases in his study of individuals with mental handicap (Penrose 1938); this was the earliest serious attempt to study the genetics of mental retardation. The condition was renamed by Dr Penrose and his colleague Dr J.H. Quastel, to be consistent with the terminology used for other inherited metabolic disorders (Alkaptonuria, Cystinuria), as **Phenylketonuria** (PKU) – i.e. due to the presence of the abnormal compound (PPA) in the **urine** being a **phenylketone** (chemical classification). PKU thus became an important early example of a genetic cause for mental retardation. Subsequent work then focussed on searching for other disorders like PKU in individuals who were in institutional care as a cause of their mental illness. In the following years many of the now well established genetic and chromosomal causes of mental deficiency were discovered. Other biochemically based disorders – which are now referred to collectively as Inherited Metabolic Disorders (IMD) – were subsequently described over the ensuing years.

Sadly all this work did not benefit the two children diagnosed by Dr Følling.

Early History of Phenylketonuria
In the immediate years the main research thrust for PKU was the study of genetics and detection of carriers, and it took a further decade for the full significance of Dr Følling's original discovery of this rare disease to be fully appreciated. More cases of PKU had continued to be reported by others and it had become clear that this was a significant cause of mental retardation in the population. This was brought to the attention of physicians by Professor Penrose's inaugural address at University College London. He summarised the characteristic clinical picture of PKU which enables a skilled observer to make a diagnosis before the urine is tested. The typical features included fair hair and often blue eyes, eczema and the peculiar mouse like smell. Those with PKU were often hyperactive and had accentuated reflexes, microcephaly (small head) and epilepsy; they were often referred to as feebleminded. Most were severely affected with 60% classified as idiots, 30% imbeciles and 10% with higher grade of mental handicap (Penrose 1946). The physical health of the individuals was generally good and they lived into adult life.

In the early part of the 20th century there was a stigma and shame associated with people with mental retardation and many were considered as hopeless cases and destined to live in institutions. The organisation of services for the care of those individuals whom we now refer to as having learning disabilities, and the description and categorisation of their severity, has been through huge changes over the duration of this story. A brief overview of this history is outlined in Appendix III including the changes in terminology. In 1951 most individuals with PKU presented as a bleak picture with no options for treatment and a life spent in asylums from their early years; it was estimated that there were 1600 such cases in Great Britain (Munro 1947). At this time it was thought that the incidence of PKU in the general population in the UK was about 1 in 50000 (Penrose 1946).

The idea that it might be important to test for PKU in younger mentally retarded children, especially those with characteristic features, was suggested and the ferric chloride test on urine began to be used in this situation. Five infants/children diagnosed with PKU (age range 18 months – 10 years) were reported by Dr Louis Woolf a chemist from Great Ormond Street Hospital, London in 1951 – the younger ones being amongst the youngest reported cases at the time (Woolf and Vulliamy 1951). Dr Woolf had tried supplementing the diet of two of these cases with glutamic acid, as a possible way of reducing blood phenylalanine level by increasing its excretion. Disappointingly the blood phenylalanine was not lowered and there was no benefit in the children's development. However this work showed that practice was beginning to turn to earlier diagnosis and importantly discussions occurring about whether there might be methods of alleviating the condition. It is important to remind ourselves that at this stage in the history of PKU a causal relationship between the abnormal chemicals found and the mental and physical abnormalities had not been established. It was only in 1953, part way through this story, when the deficiency of the enzyme phenylalanine hydroxylase (PAH) as the cause of PKU was confirmed in the liver by George Jervis in the United States (Jervis 1953).

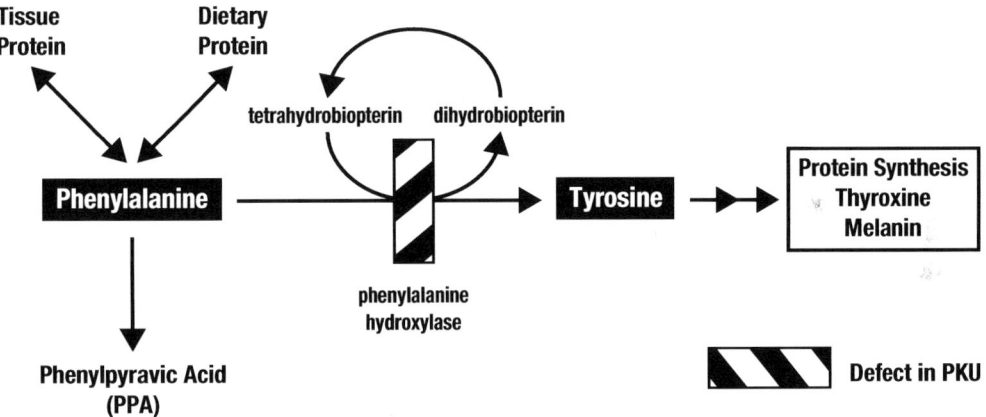

Phenylalanine metabolism showing defect in PKU.

The enzyme PAH requires a catalyst (cofactor) – tetrahydrobiopterin. The importance and significance of tetrahydrobiopterin became appreciated much later in understanding the different types of PKU (p.109).

4

SHEILA – DIAGNOSIS

Dr Hickmans: 'The RMO (Resident Medical Officer) came to us and said he had a mentally backward child whose urine gave olive-green colour with ferric chloride and that it might be a PKU'.

The Ferric Chloride Test
The ferric chloride testing of urine from patients with mental retardation had been introduced into the Birmingham clinic by Dr Bickel in 1951. He had learnt about this testing whilst working with Professor Fanconi in Zurich prior to his arrival in Birmingham. During this time Professor Fanconi, one morning on his 7.30am ward round, had asked Dr Bickel *'Why did they not test their retarded patients for PKU?'* – he had only read about this test that same morning and was obviously an early riser. Dr Bickel had remembered this event and so to impress his new colleague, Dr Gerrard, he had asked the very same question at BCH. *'Why do you not test the retarded patients for PKU?'* It was soon introduced to the Birmingham clinic (Bickel 1996).

Mary had brought a sample of Sheila's urine to the outpatient clinic where it was tested by placing a few drops of the ferric chloride reagent into the urine. It quickly turned the characteristic olive-green colour, described by Dr Følling. Sheila was only the third patient they had tested. Can you imagine the Doctors' response at this finding? This must be PKU and would be their first case!

We don't know how soon Mary was informed about the finding or what she was told about what it might mean for her daughter. However, it was clear that the doctors were excited and arranged to admit Sheila to the Children's Hospital a few months later to confirm their finding and further investigate her. They sent a letter to the family doctor, Dr Allin saying: *'Sheila suffers from phenylpyruvic oligophrenia. As far as we know no line of treatment is of any avail, but we will admit her to hospital in a month or two for further investigation'.* Sheila continued to live at home in Matlock Road for the next few months until her hospital admission. Terry and Trevor were now six and three years of age. This must have been an anxious time for Mary knowing that the doctors had found something abnormal with Sheila's urine but wondering what it all meant.

4. Sheila – Diagnosis

First Hospital Admission

Sheila was admitted to Birmingham Children's Hospital under the care of Dr Smellie on 25th September 1951, now aged almost two years. The admission had been organised in order to undertake more detailed investigations i.e. to confirm the initial finding from the positive ferric chloride test on her urine that she had PKU. Mary would have taken Sheila from their home in Matlock Road (see Map Birmingham, 4) by bus, with a change of bus in the city centre, to the hospital at Ladywood on the west side of the city (see Map Birmingham, 6). It must have been a frightening prospect for Mary to leave Sheila alone in the hospital ward for the first time and we can imagine how worried she must have been for her daughter.

The hospital in the 1950s was organised with long nightingale style wards, with children of all ages from young infants like Sheila to adolescents with a variety of illnesses. Nurses wore rather severe uniforms, especially the ward sister and matron. To a little two year old girl this must have been scary. Visiting hours were very limited and visiting had only recently been allowed since the end of the war; during the war parents were excluded from contact with their child (Waterhouse, 1962). The object of these strict rules was to prevent infection and

Ward at BCH c.1950.

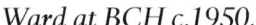

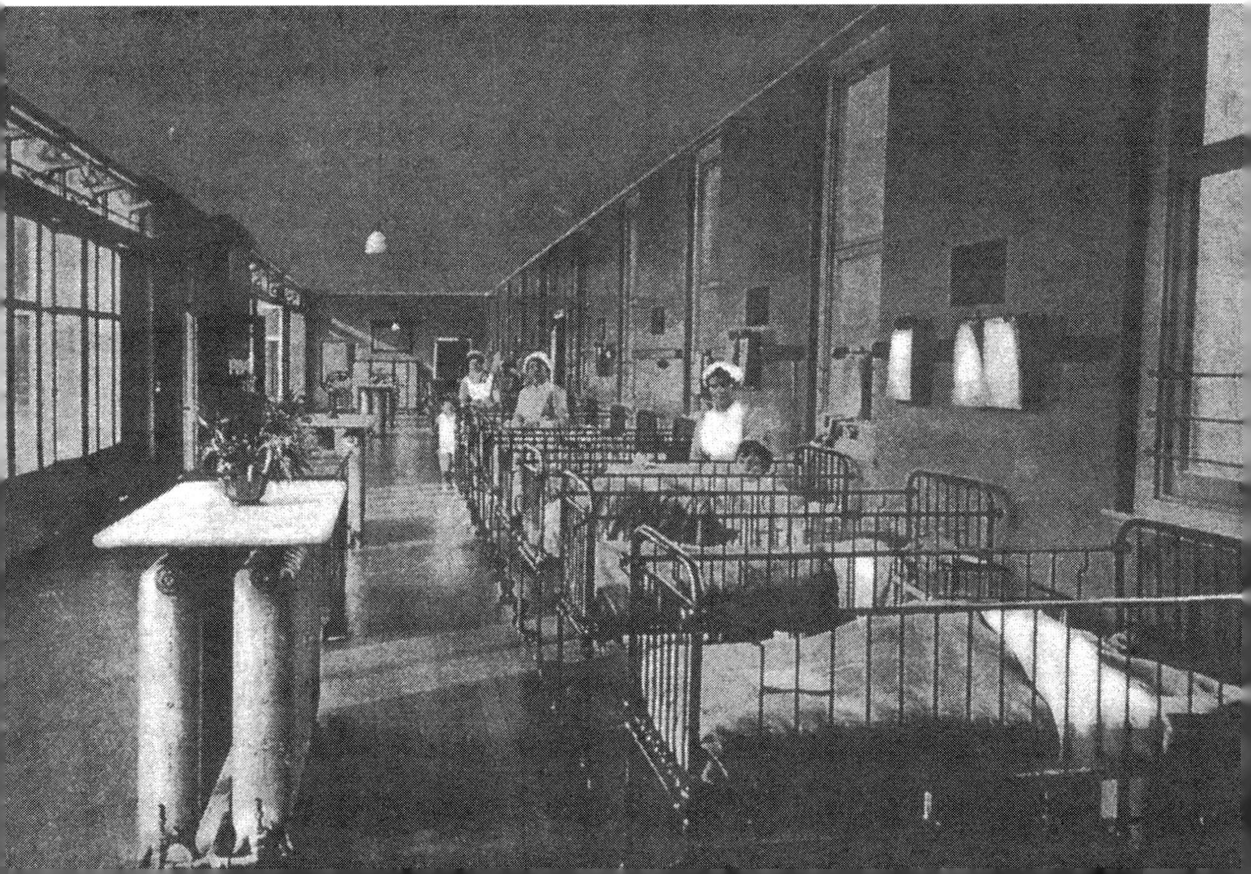

to avoid emotional distress. Once it was realised that far greater problems might be created with the continuation of this system things changed, and from July 1948 parents were allowed to visit for an hour, once a fortnight but only after a child had been in hospital for two weeks. After a trial period this was made a permanent arrangement and continued until 1952. Subsequently further relaxation occurred to allow an hour of visiting on Sundays, or as an alternative an hour during the week, but only if the ward sister gave permission. In 1953 daily visiting began. During this initial admission Sheila must have missed her Mum, been homesick and longing for her Mum to come – when Mary did come for the fortnightly visit it was for such a short length of time. We assume children were not allowed to visit in 1951 and certainly Terry and Trevor have no recollection of visiting their sister at this time.

On admission Sheila, at two years of age, was unable to sit for long (she did not sit without support until she was 18 months of age), could not stand without support and could neither walk nor talk. She showed no interest in food or her surroundings and lay in her cot moaning and crying for hours, banging her head or rolling it from side to side to such an extent that her hair was nearly worn off at the back and sides. Her hair was fair and described by Dr Hickmans as like '***tow***'* (see Appendix IV, set 1). Sheila continued to have a frequent rocking motion and her movements were generally exaggerated. She was well-nourished but had some rough skin and eczema; there were no other abnormal physical signs; she had a musty 'mouse like' smell. These were the characteristic symptoms of PKU described by Dr Fölling and others. The biochemical investigations to confirm the suspected diagnosis of PKU were undertaken on blood and urine in Dr Hickmans' laboratory.

*****tow*** *is an Old English word derived from spinning. It is defined as: i.the coarse and broken part of flax or hemp prepared for spinning ii. a bundle of untwisted natural or man-made fibres.*

Specimen Collection
Specimen collection would not have been easy. Very few methods were in existence at that time for measuring chemicals in blood that were suitable for babies and young infants and would require inappropriately large volumes for a two year old. Each test was usually done in duplicate and would have required as much as 10ml blood – this compares to methods today which use only a 10μl volume – a thousand times less. 10ml blood would have been a large amount to take from a little girl on repeated occasions over many weeks, considering her total blood volume would be in the order of 800ml. Laboratory methods were very

labour intensive. For blood this usually involved a preliminary process to remove proteins before the specific chemical could be measured. Urine collection would also have been very difficult. Sheila was incontinent and was kept on a special metabolic bed which had apparatus attached for collecting the urine. Urine would be collected on a continual basis over a period of time (referred to as a 'timed urine'), often over a whole day. Imagine how difficult this would have been for a two year girl to endure as 24 hour urine collections were obtained, not just once but several times, day after day. During the collection period the urine was kept refrigerated with a preservative and when completed was stored deep frozen at -10°C before being thawed prior to analysis in the biochemistry laboratory.

5

THE BIOCHEMISTRY LABORATORY

BCH Annual Report 1922: 'The committee of management realises that upon chemical and bacteriological research modern medicine is built' (Waterhouse 1962).

General Laboratory and Staffing

Evelyn Hickmans had established the laboratory in 1923. Initially located in a small room adjacent to ward 6 in the main hospital the laboratory moved into larger rooms in the basement of the new outpatient building in 1925. The staff increased with a second biochemist and a research student. In the mid-1930s the laboratory was again relocated to an even larger area with museum and library attached, with separate rooms for balances, washing up of bottles and equipment – in fact it was quite spacious. It formed an extension to the Pathology (Histopathology) laboratory. This early laboratory at BCH with (presumed) staff (all female) is pictured below.

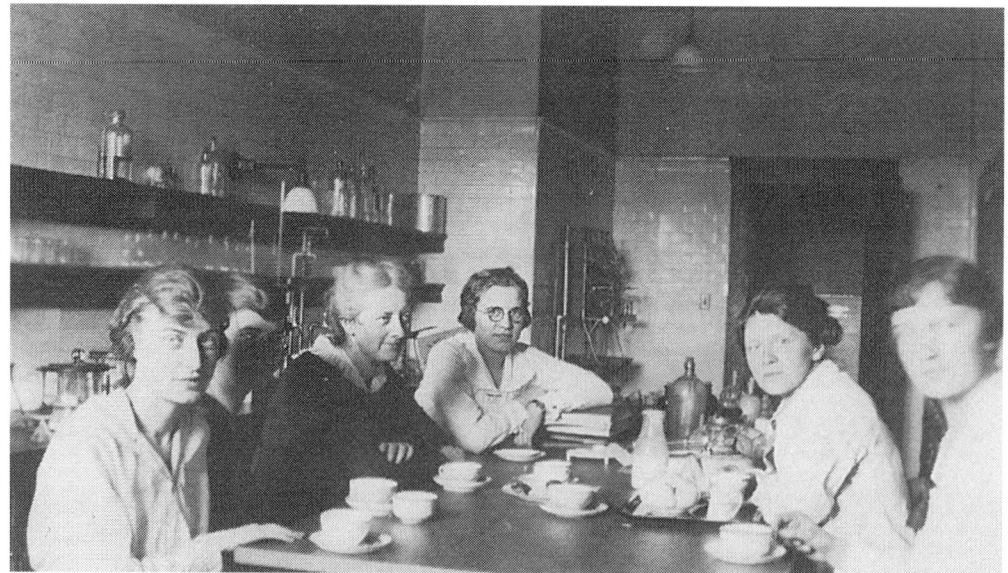

Tea Party in Early Biochemistry Laboratory BCH.

5. The Biochemistry Laboratory

Two other notable biochemists, also from Wolverhampton, Miss Ethel Finch M.Sc. and Miss Eva Tonks M.Sc., both graduate chemists from Birmingham University, worked with Evelyn Hickmans in these early years. A 'new' two storey laboratory block was built around the late 1940s and this is probably where Horst Bickel came to work at the start of his PhD in 1949.

Tom Day was a young biochemistry student who had gone to study Biochemistry at Birmingham University in 1948; in his final year his then Professor, Peter Gilding, arranged for him and another student to work at one of the local hospitals to get some experience in a 'real' laboratory. There were two possibilities: the General hospital and the Children's hospital. The two students tossed a coin and Tom started in October 1950 in Dr Hickmans' laboratory. His recollection is of the laboratory being in a building separate from the main hospital on the second floor. As a young student he remembers Evelyn Hickmans as a small but formidable lady – rather *'elderly and getting on a bit'* (she was in fact 68 years of age) in the eyes of a 20 year old. *'She arrived every morning with a large leather bag and went to her office, but only after she had huffed and puffed and slammed all the windows closed saying there was too much fresh air!'* Tom had usually opened the windows because it was stuffy and full of smells and fumes. Apart from Brian Rudd, a junior laboratory assistant at the time, the rest of the small staff were female. He and Brian formed a close friendship as they went down to the pub at lunchtime and shared a *'woodbine'* cigarette between them as their lunch. His recollection of his time at BCH was of always *'getting into trouble'*, and he wasn't sure if Dr Hickmans liked having the *'boys'* in her laboratory. We felt *'we were there under sufferance'*.

The other three workers in the general laboratory at that time were Sheila, Joan, and Patricia Hughes who subsequently became a Consultant Biochemist at Exeter Hospital. A small repertoire of general chemical tests were undertaken on blood, urine and faeces. The more common assays comprised blood sugar, urea (for kidney function) and bilirubin (to assess jaundice and liver disease) and were undertaken by simple colour reactions. This involved visual comparison of the depth of colour produced in a test tube by the test specimen with that of known standards of the compound (a Lovibond Comparator was used). Apart from a centrifuge there were no laboratory instruments as we know them today. There were about 30-40 tests done each day and some would take 2-3 days to complete. This compares to a present day workload in 2019 of approximately 3500 tests (600 specimens)* per day, most of which are completed within a matter of hours.

In addition to these general assays, a major part of the work was identifying the amino acids in blood and urine using chromatography, this was done in a separate room on the same floor and immediately adjacent to the general laboratory. Other special tests set up to help with Sheila's diagnosis and treatment included phenylpyruvic acid measured in urine, also using a chromatographic method (Penrose and Quastel 1937). Microbiological assays were used to measure phenylalanine and tyrosine (Henderson and Snell 1948).

When Tom arrived at BCH in 1950, he was asked to help a young German doctor with the chromatography work – Dr Horst Bickel (see profile p17). Tom recalls being told by Dr Hickmans:

'I haven't got time to teach you any general biochemistry – we don't need anyone to do any general work, we are fully staffed. We have a German doctor here, Horst Bickel and he would be very pleased if you would help him'.

Dr Bickel had been at BCH for about two years working on amino acid chromatography as part of his PhD and had an assistant Anne Whitehouse, whom Tom subsequently married. Tom learnt how to do the chromatography and undertook a lot of the amino acid work during his time there. This was the year when Sheila was diagnosed and no doubt Tom helped, together with Anne, with the many analyses on specimens from Sheila.

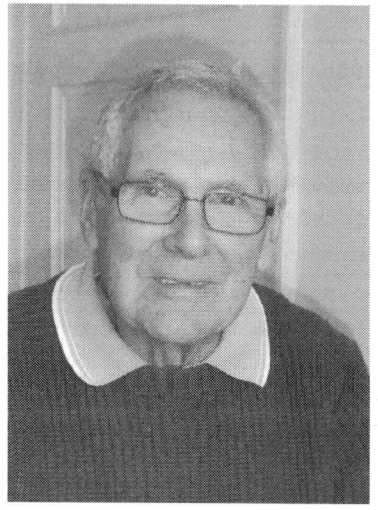

Tom Day at his home in Colchester, UK 2018.

*Data courtesy of Mary Anne Preece, Clinical Chemistry Department, BCH 2019.

Amino Acid Chromatography

There are 20 'common' amino acids in human blood and urine which can be separated and identified using partition chromatography, a technique developed for use on paper for biological fluids by Charles Dent at University College, London in the late 1940s. The technique had been set up at BCH in Dr Hickmans' laboratory.

The method involves placing a small amount of the prepared body fluid on one corner of the paper and allowing it to be carried in a solvent (usually a mixture of different chemicals) across the paper. The different amino acids in the fluid, owing to their different chemical properties, are carried across the paper by the solvent at different rates. The paper is then dried and further separation of the amino acids is achieved with a second solvent which is allowed to travel across the paper at right angles to the original. This allows the different amino acids to separate into a reproducible and characteristic pattern. They are then visualised with a stain (usually ninhydrin) which colours them a range of colours – blue, purple, pink, grey or yellow. Each individual amino acid is identified by its location and colour. The colour intensity and size of the 'spot' can be used to estimate the quantity. For reproducible results chromatography requires a stable room temperature and an atmosphere saturated with the solvent. A 'map' (chromatogram) to show location of each amino acid is then produced.

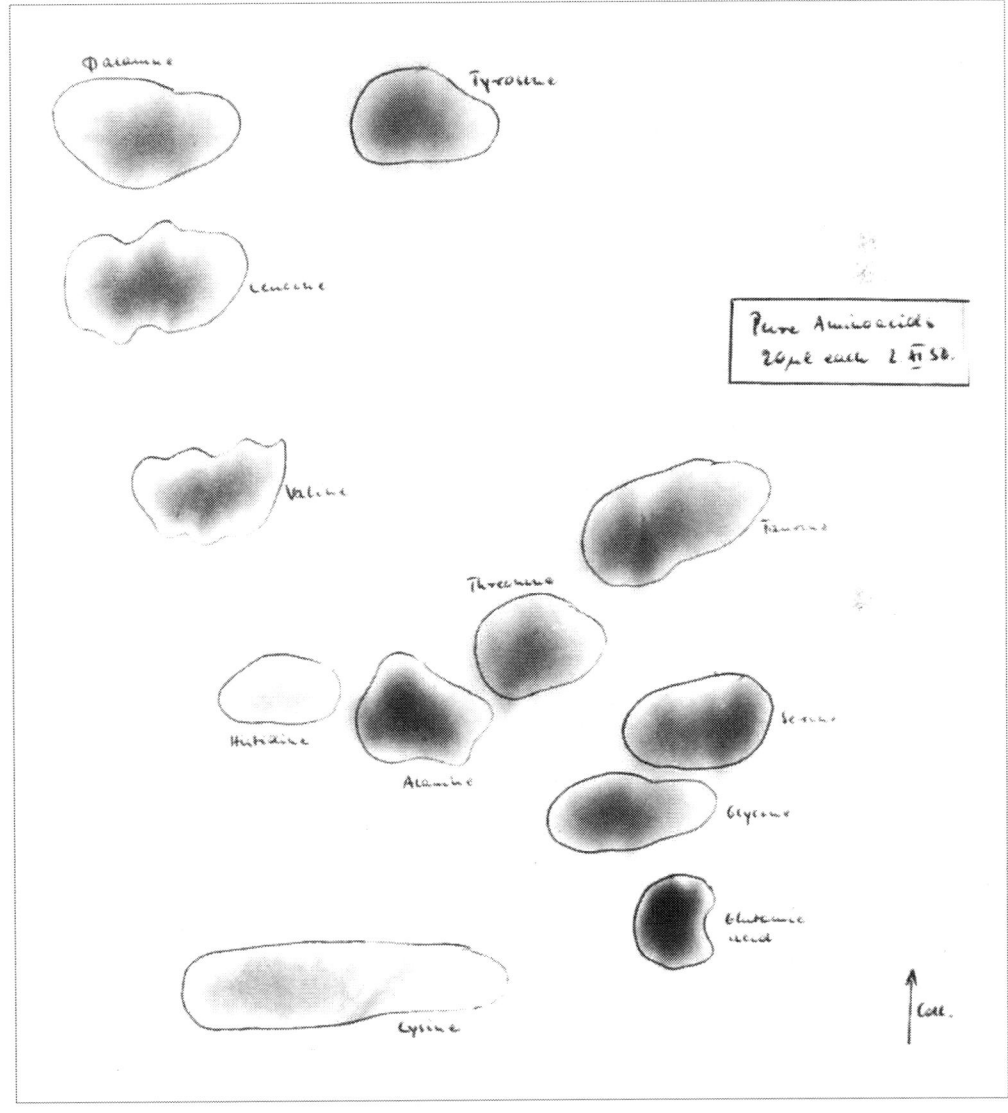

Chromatogram of pure amino acids (reproduced from Bickel, H. 1952).

The illustration (p.31) shows the separation of a mixture of pure amino acids using chromatography, obtained by Dr Bickel at BCH.

These chromatographic methods were very labour intensive. Tom Day describes the large glass chromatography tanks for the solvent and the large sheets of paper, approximately 2ft x 1ft (60.96cm x 30.48cm), which were used. It was necessary to load a quantity of urine with a certain 'standardized' nitrogen content, to allow for different urine concentrations, and so the first job was to analyse the nitrogen content of each urine. One of Tom's regular jobs was to undertake these total nitrogen assays on every urine and it took him all day. A calculated volume of each urine had then to be very carefully layered onto a separate sheet of the thick chromatography paper ('blotting paper') in as small an area as possible, allowing it to dry between each application. Each amino acid was 'quantified' by comparison of the intensity of its colour with standards of a pure amino acid on the same paper.

The solvents used for the chromatography contained phenol, a noxious chemical which burned the skin if in contact. There were no protective gloves, no eye cover and no fume extraction – unimaginable today with current safety regulations. Tom remembers the lab being *'thick with chemicals'* – hence his passion to keep opening the windows. Other constituents of the amino acid solvent mix were lutidine and collidine which Dr Hickmans obtained from the Yorkshire Tar Distillers. They are products of coal tar distillation and now known to be highly toxic but, like so many accepted laboratory practices in those times, considered of little consequence. In Tom's words at over 80 years of age *'it never did us any harm!'* The ninhydrin stain was not without its mark on the laboratory worker as with no protective gloves it was impossible not to end up with dark purple finger tips which did not wash off.

Tom described how after undertaking the total nitrogen analysis the urine was spotted on the paper in the afternoon, and the chromatography with the first solvent conducted overnight. Next morning the paper would be dried and then the process repeated overnight with the second solvent. The following day the paper would be dried again and then, after spaying with ninhydrin, was allowed to develop the colours overnight. The following morning *'we would look at the coloured spots, and discuss with Dr Bickel'*. The whole process took three days and in Dr Hickmans words: *'three of us worked day and night on chromatograms otherwise we would never have got the work done; it required a dark room, steady temperature and very careful spotting'* (see Appendix IV, set 5).

A chromatography room was still in use at BCH in the 1970s and 1980s. It was a dingy, claustrophobic and miserable room almost in total darkness and separated from the main laboratory block close to the engineers' department and hospital boiler room. It had no exhaust system, only windows for ventilation and

5. The Biochemistry Laboratory

the 'air' was 'thick with chemicals'. There were large cabinets for drying the chromatograms and huge floor-standing glass tanks. By 1970 little had changed in the methodology since the 1950s.

Dr Bickel's PhD

The topic of Horst Bickel's PhD at BCH was the systematic study of urine amino acids in children, to ascertain the normal pattern and variation in pathological conditions. Using paper chromatography he investigated 290 healthy children/infants and 292 with various disease states, including five cases of PKU. It involved preparation of over 5100 chromatograms undertaken between 1949 and 1952 with the help of Tom, Brian and Anne. Dr Bickel obtained his PhD from Birmingham University in 1953 and in it he wrote the following acknowledgment: *'my special thanks are due to Dr Evelyn Hickmans, to her assistants in the Biochemical Department and to B Rudd (Brian), technical assistant whose tireless and reliable work has greatly assisted this study'.*

Tom remembers Horst Bickel very fondly:

'He was a very nice chap, of course he was very young in those days. He was a Medical Officer in the German navy in the U boat section – but I'm not sure if he actually went in U boats!' Others have also mentioned that he was on a U boat during the war but it is now clear that this story was 'invented' – probably by his colleagues in Birmingham as a bit of mischief making – or maybe Horst Bickel himself started the rumour! (See profile of Horst Bickel p.17)

Tom:

'He never talked about life as it was so soon after the war. Some people were a bit suspicious of him but in the scientific community it didn't matter. He was keen on tennis and used to play tennis with the lady who became my wife. He was often in the lab – he spent a lot of time in the lab'.

After leaving BCH in late 1951 Tom went to work at Birmingham Women's Hospital until 1955 before

Dr Bickel's PhD undertaken at BCH (reproduced from Bickel, H. 1952).

continuing his career in Clinical Biochemistry, becoming a Consultant Biochemist at Colchester Hospital, Essex. Brian Rudd went on to do a degree and PhD at Birmingham University and had a long and successful career in Clinical Chemistry, specialising as a Consultant Clinical Scientist in Endocrinology in Birmingham. Anne Whitehouse went on to study Pharmacy and married Tom. Tom, Anne and Brian at the time played a significant part of the Sheila Jones story, although unaware at the time that their work with Horst Bickel and Evelyn Hickmans would become part of this important piece of medical history.

6

SHEILA – CONFIRMATION OF THE DIAGNOSIS

Dr Bickel: 'The mother of course was in despair and could not share our excitement about the rare diagnosis, nor our interest in the strong phenylalanine spot on the chromatogram'.

PKU Confirmed
In September 1951 Sheila's diagnosis of PKU was confirmed by detecting large amounts of phenylalanine in her blood and urine. At least two chromatograms of each specimen were prepared and compared with several test spots of known amounts of a pure amino acid chromatographed at the same time under identical conditions. In this way the size and intensity of the purple spot of phenylalanine on Sheila's chromatogram could be compared with the standard spots and an assessment made of their amount. Sheila's plasma phenylalanine level was far in excess of amounts seen in infants without PKU, with a level approximately 40 times normal, and her tyrosine level about half the amount seen in normal infants. Phenylpyruvic acid levels were greatly increased. This pattern of abnormalities fitted with the metabolic block described in PKU (see p.23) so there was no doubt about Sheila's diagnosis. During this admission, her two brothers and mother were also tested and no excess phenylalanine or phenylpyruvic acid was found in their urines. Sheila's father was unavailable for testing.

Mary's Persistence
The doctors at Birmingham were very excited about their diagnosis, with Dr Bickel proudly showing Mary Jones *'my beautiful paper chromatogram'* with the very strong phenylalanine spot proving the diagnosis of PKU. But this did not help Mary or Sheila as there was no treatment established for PKU. Those diagnosed with PKU at this time were severely mentally impaired. Early research work since the discovery of the disorder had concentrated on understanding the inheritance of PKU, working out the metabolic pathway and developing methods for its diagnosis. It must have been difficult for Mary to understand what the

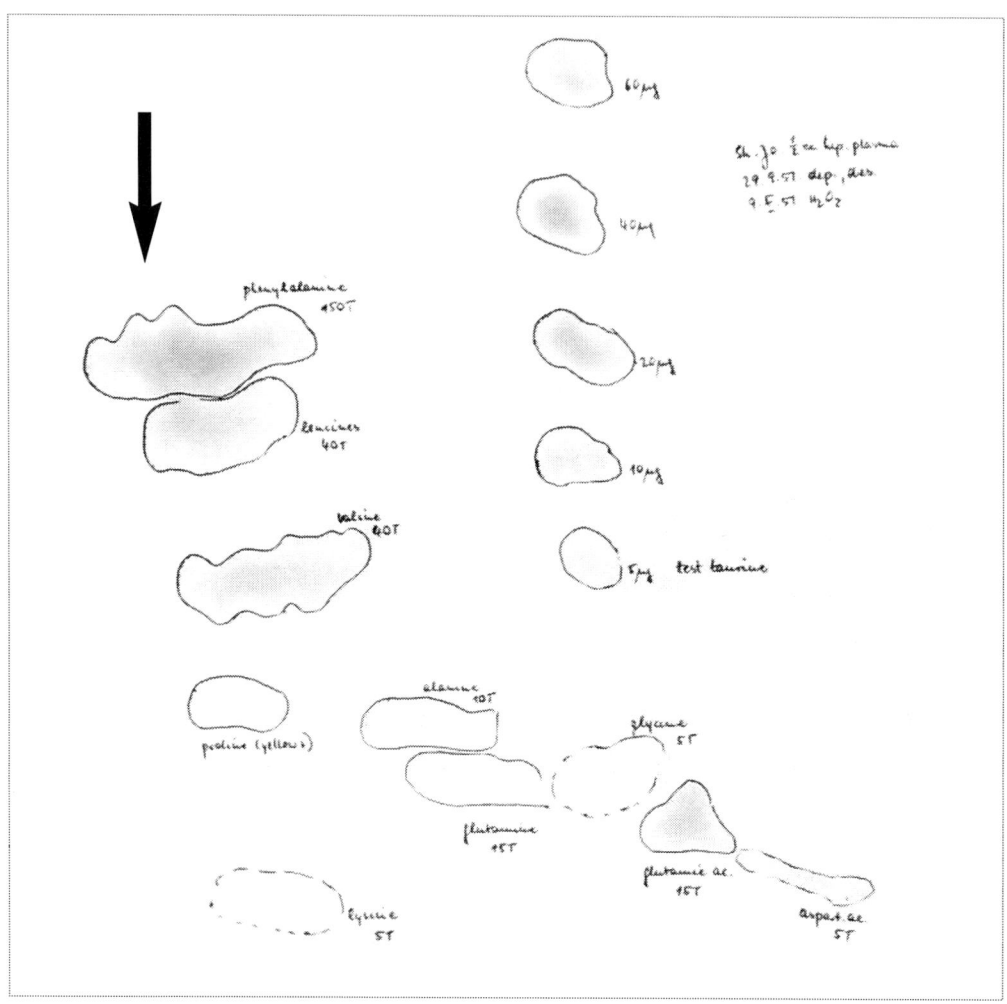

Chromatogram of amino acids in plasma from Sheila at diagnosis – note the strong phenylalanine spot indicated with arrow (reproduced from Bickel, H. 1952).

disorder was and why the doctors were so excited. What was PKU? How might the condition progress? What did this mean for Sheila? Mary could see that Sheila was not normal like her two boys and must have known that the future did not look good for her daughter. Why could the doctors not treat Sheila? Mary was desperate; she wanted help for Sheila and would not take no for an answer.

Dr Bickel: 'Instead she waited for me every morning before the laboratory door, making quite clear it was treatment what she wanted for her child, not fancy investigations. She did not accept that so far there was no therapy for this condition. The

6. Sheila – Confirmation of the Diagnosis

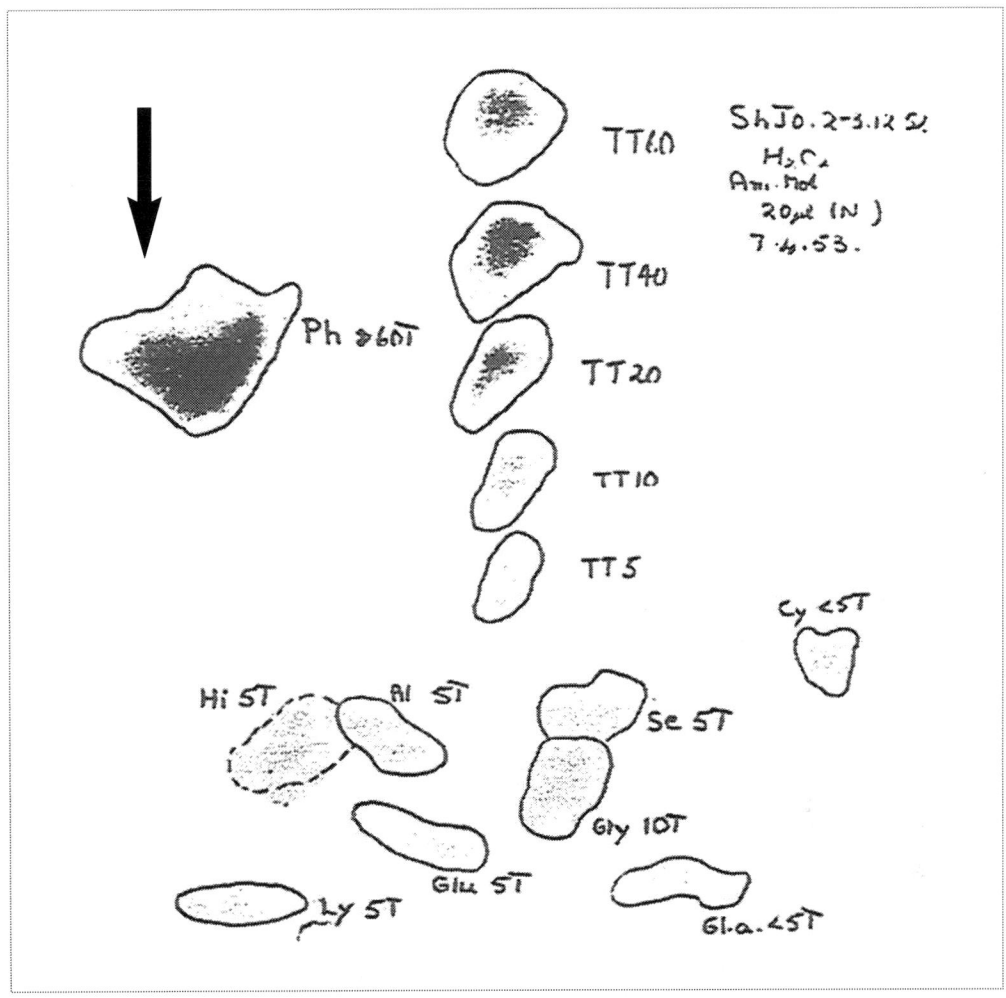

Chromatogram of amino acids in urine from Sheila showing excess phenylalanine indicated with arrow (reproduced from Bickel, H. et al 1954).

mother's perseverance gave me no chance to rest on the strength of a fine diagnosis' (see Appendix IV, set 4).

It seems likely that this plea and pestering of Dr Bickel occurred on several occasions whilst Sheila was in hospital and presumably when Mary was visiting Sheila on the ward during the September/October admission. One can imagine Mary coming from the ward to stand outside the laboratory block to 'catch' Dr Bickel as he went to his work there. Who looked after Terry and Trevor whilst Mary was visiting Sheila in hospital? Maybe they were at school or being looked after by the lodgers or neighbours? They can't remember anything about this – they were very young.

Dr Bickel has described on numerous occasions that it was Mary's demands and persistence in asking for treatment for her daughter which then pushed him and Dr Hickmans to look at what might be possible as a treatment. '**When are you going to treat my child?**' was the plea from Mary. When Dr Bickel explained there was no treatment available the response from Mary was '**can't you find one?**' There was no quick solution. How could they find a way to treat Sheila?

Dr Bickel mentioned in his PhD thesis that tyrosine deficiency had been suggested as a possible cause of the mental retardation in PKU but this hypothesis lacked confirmation; a few patients had been given tyrosine by others but this had not produced any improvement in their mental condition. Under the pressure from Mary, Dr Bickel with his co-workers Dr Gerrard and Dr Hickmans wondered, as others had previously, if there might be a relationship between Sheila's condition and the phenylalanine excess in her body fluids. Would removal of phenylalanine in her diet be a possibility?

After the admission to confirm her diagnosis of PKU Sheila was then discharged home to Matlock Road on 11th October 1951; she had been in hospital just over two weeks but Mary's persistence had paid off – the doctors had been persuaded by Mary to see if they could find a treatment for Sheila. Mary would however have to wait another seven weeks whilst the doctors set about their plans to see if they could make a special diet which they could try. This must have been a very anxious time for Mary not knowing what might be possible and what the future was for Sheila?

7

SHEILA'S TREATMENT 1951-1953

*Dr Bickel described how 'he and Dr Hickmans became
as black as coal miners as they prepared the formula'.*

Diet Preparation
The idea of a diet as a possible form of treatment for PKU was not new. Lionel Penrose had speculated that if phenylalanine could be removed from the diet then maybe the disorder could be treated, but how was this to be done? Phenylalanine is a constituent of all dietary protein, each different protein (e.g. from milk, eggs, meat, fish) being about equally rich in phenylalanine. Phenylalanine is necessary for protein synthesis to enable normal growth and development. Humans cannot produce it so they must obtain it from the foods they eat and it is therefore referred to as an 'essential' amino acid. Only part of the ingested phenylalanine is required for the synthesis of new proteins, the remainder normally being converted to the amino acid tyrosine. As phenylalanine is found in almost all foods, except pure carbohydrates and fats, it had seemed to be impossible from the early discussions to produce a nutritionally adequate diet based on this idea. There was also some scepticism about whether the biochemical abnormality was in fact the cause of the mental retardation in PKU. This early idea from the 1930s had therefore not progressed and the prospect of a dietary therapy had seemed remote.

When re-visiting the idea in 1951, the Birmingham doctors considered how they could remove phenylalanine from Sheila's diet. Two possibilities had been considered as an alternative to natural protein; formulation of a mixture of pure l-amino acids (excluding phenylalanine) in appropriate amounts or the removal of phenylalanine from a natural protein source. The former idea would be very expensive as it would be necessary to purchase the individual l-amino acids, and the estimated costs were felt to be prohibitive. A chemical method for removal of phenylalanine from natural protein had been used in the USA for work unrelated to PKU (Block and Bolling 1951). Phenylalanine had been removed from a mixture of amino acids (produced from the breakdown of a natural protein) by passing through a column of activated charcoal – charcoal is adsorbent and selectively binds certain molecules, in this case the aromatic amino acids, including phenylalanine. This idea had been taken further by Louis Woolf (see p.23), working at Great Ormond Street Hospital, London. He had suggested that it might be possible to treat those with PKU with a diet in which the phenylalanine had been removed in this same way, by using charcoal, and the resulting mixture then being used as a substitute for natural protein. Dr Woolf had already had experience of breaking down (hydrolysing) milk protein (casein) into constituent amino acids as a product to treat those with malnutrition during the aftermath of the WWII. The next step would be to remove the phenylalanine. He had been trying to convince his medical colleagues in London to try a diet low in phenylalanine, produced in this way for PKU, but they had not been prepared to do this. Dr Bickel and Dr Hickmans, when searching for possible treatment for Sheila, were aware of Dr Woolf's expertise and he very generously shared his ideas with them. Dr Woolf explained how they might go about producing such a diet, and with his help the team at BCH then set about it. The plan was to prepare a phenylalanine free product from a casein hydrolysate, using activated charcoal, and this would be done in Dr Hickmans' laboratory. This was a ground breaking step.

Allen and Hanburys, a British pharmaceutical company, were already producing casein hydrolysate to treat individuals with malnutrition after World War II and the initial hydrolysate used by Dr Bickel and Dr Hickmans was obtained from them as a gift for 'research'. The phenylalanine would then be removed from this hydrolysate by treating with activated charcoal (Scramm and Primosigh 1943; Tiselius 1947).

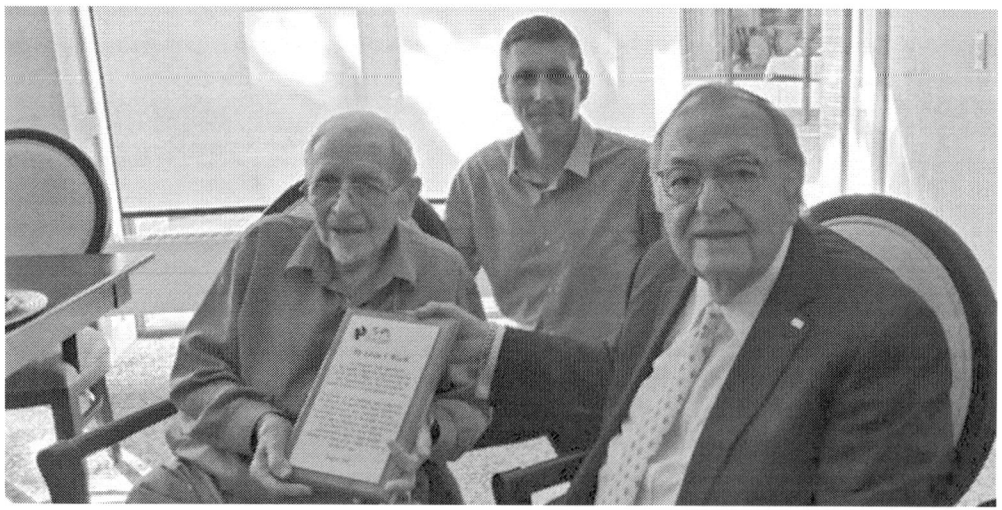

Dr Louis Woolf celebrating his 100th birthday 2019. From left to right: Dr Louis Woolf, Dr Graham Sinclair and Professor Rodney Howell (photograph courtesy of Professor Rodney Howell, ISNS).

The chemical process removes not just phenylalanine but also tyrosine and tryptophan (the aromatic amino acids) from the others. The first stage was to mix a 10% solution of the hydrolysed casein in acetic acid with acidified charcoal. This was done by stirring together in a glass beaker for an hour, and repeating a couple of times. The resulting solution was then allowed to slowly flow through a glass column containing charcoal to complete the removal of the phenylalanine. The original glass column used in 1951 to prepare the diet for Sheila was 3ft long x 2ins diameter (91.5cm x 5cm) and is on display in the current Clinical Chemistry Department at BCH. The charcoal used to fill the column was a black powder and the resulting solution (filtrate) emerging from the bottom of the column resembled strong tea in appearance – it was a strong acid solution. This was done repeatedly

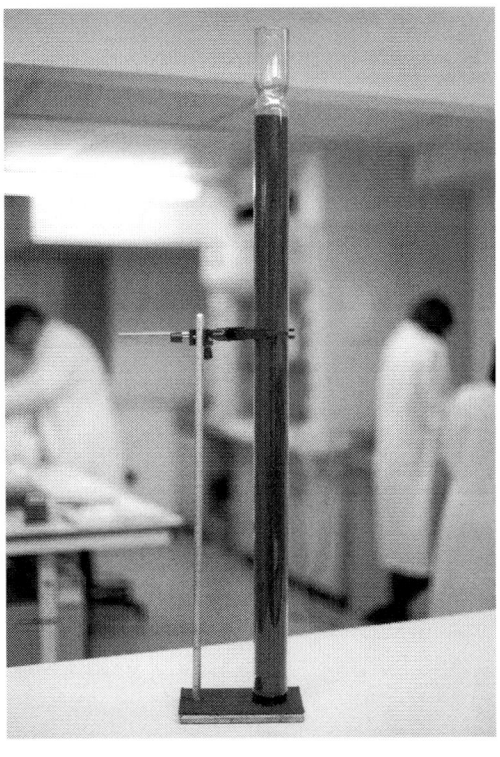

Charcoal column used to prepare Sheila's Special Mixture.

several times until the resulting filtrate from the column had no detectable phenylalanine, this was checked by seeing if it would enable growth of a special bacterium which required phenylalanine to grow.

The resulting mixture from the column was a solution of the individual amino acids from the broken down casein but free from phenylalanine and the other amino acids which had also been removed by the adsorption process. The filtrate from the column was also tested using amino acid chromatography which showed that tyrosine, tryptophan and cystine had also been removed in addition to phenylalanine. The resulting filtrate solution was then made up to a final volume which had been calculated to be equivalent to 1g protein; this was the basis for Sheila's diet to replace her natural protein – this final solution was the 'special mixture' or formula.

The process for producing this mixture was difficult and time consuming and had to be done in a cold room or it would deteriorate and be useless as a food. The charcoal got on everything and as they prepared the formula (Appendix V;

Gerrard 1962) the sight of Dr Bickel wrapped in layers of sweaters, topped by a charcoal smudged lab coat became a common sight at the hospital. Dr Bickel distinctly remembered having to work in the freezing laboratory whilst his family enjoyed a warm Christmas celebration without him (Koch 1997).

Dr Gerrard subsequently recounted in 1962 (see Appendix V, p.150): *'Block had said it would certainly be possible to prepare a suitable formula – or food – using activated charcoal, but when later confronted with the news that this had actually been done in Birmingham, he said that though he knew it had been theoretically possible he had always thought it would have been quite impracticable'.*

Second Admission to BCH

After many weeks of working in the laboratory during the autumn of 1951 enough of the 'mixture' had been prepared and so Sheila was admitted for a second time, on 21st November 1951, in order to begin a trial of the dietary treatment. You can imagine the excitement from the doctors as they embarked on this, although not without some concern of what effects it might produce for Sheila. Would she take the diet? Would there be any harmful effects? This had never been tried before. This was completely unknown territory. The impact for the nurses on the ward would have been significant with 24 hour urine collections to supervise and the need to give Sheila this unusual, restrictive and unpleasant diet. We subsequently know from her brothers what a struggle it was to give Sheila this mixture and this must have been the situation whilst she was in hospital.

How would Mary have been feeling? What would this treatment do to her daughter? There must have been many different emotions; apprehension, hope, and fear. She badly wanted treatment for Sheila and had the courage to let the doctors try something new, but these must have been anxious days and weeks. It would eventually involve a long stay in hospital for Sheila with all the consequent ramifications for the family with visits to the hospital, not least of which was the need to find the money for the bus fares. Mary had two young sons at home to look after. She was on her own – there was no one to help her. It was a huge commitment as she embarked on the treatment for her daughter.

Phenylalanine Free Diet

The first stage of the treatment was to give Sheila a phenylalanine **free** diet, with her only source of protein being the special mixture i.e. the acid casein hydrolysate after removal of the phenylalanine (protein substitute). There was no natural protein for Sheila – no milk, fish, eggs or meat. The necessary minerals, vitamins, fats and carbohydrates, in pure form, were added to try and ensure a nutritionally adequate diet. Tryptophan and cystine, as they had been lost in preparation of the mixture were added as pure amino acids. The resulting formula would have been extremely unpleasant, especially for a two year old. The amount of this phenylalanine free mixture ingested daily was equivalent to approximately 10g protein and the diet provided about 1,100 calories per day. On 27th November, six days after her admission, Sheila started this diet with blood and urine phenylalanine levels being measured on a frequent basis as a means of monitoring the biochemical effects. The laboratory work was now going at full pelt with preparation of Sheila's diet to keep up production of a daily supply of the special mix and undertaking the numerous investigations on her blood and urine. Evelyn Hickmans, Horst Bickel, Brian Rudd, and the laboratory team were working non-stop.

A few days later Sheila's plasma and urine phenylalanine fell to normal levels, urine phenylpyruvic acid level also dropped and the ferric chloride test became negative. This was all very encouraging. The diet was having the effect on the biochemistry of her PKU that the team had hoped for. During this initial stage the tyrosine intake had also been restricted (as tyrosine had been removed by the charcoal treatment) and after five days plasma tyrosine levels, which had been low to start with, were no longer measurable and there was great concern. Sheila had rapidly lost weight. Pure tyrosine, which would have been purchased as a chemical was then added as a supplement to the diet. The effect was a prompt increase of blood tyrosine levels and weight loss was temporarily halted. After three weeks of being on the formula (now with added tyrosine) blood and urine phenylalanine levels and urine phenylpyruvic acid began to rise again. During this time there had been no immediate change in her clinical state but Sheila slowly and steadily continued to lose weight and seemed unwell; she began to vomit more frequently and was upset. She developed a generalised increase in the amino acids in her urine, findings which suggested that Sheila was beginning to break down her own body protein and that this was due to phenylalanine deficiency. Her clinical and biochemical situation had gone from one extreme to another – too much phenylalanine and now insufficient to maintain growth. The diet was having an adverse effect and clearly this regime could not continue. Sheila had become sick. This must have been very worrying for the doctors, and for Mary seeing her daughter so unwell with a diet she had hoped would make her better. Something needed to change. The question of whether they should abandon the plan for Sheila's treatment must have been considered.

Phenylalanine Reduced Diet

It was now three weeks since the diet had been started. It was clear that this mix with no phenylalanine was nutritionally inadequate and that Sheila needed some phenylalanine in order to prevent the breakdown of her own body protein and enable her to grow. Initially it was decided to add 0.8g phenylalanine daily to her diet in the form of 500ml natural milk. This commenced on 18th December, 3 weeks after starting the treatment. After this change the phenylalanine levels in blood and urine and urine phenylpyruvic acid levels began to rise, but they were still well below those at diagnosis whilst Sheila was on a normal diet with no phenylalanine restriction. This was encouraging and suggested that the mixture was now having the hoped for effect of lowering the blood chemicals which might be damaging Sheila's brain, whilst still allowing her to grow. Slowly over many weeks Sheila began to regain her lost weight on this modified regime with a low rather than no phenylalanine intake of 300-400ml milk. Progress was being made. The special mix continued to be produced by the laboratory team so Sheila could continue on the diet whilst staying in hospital to allow clinical supervision and biochemical monitoring. Sheila's weight became stable and she then began to slightly gain weight. This continued until March 1952. During this long period in hospital Terry and Trevor both remember going with their Mum to visit Sheila. Mary visited whenever possible, whilst continuing to look after Terry and Trevor at home and bearing in mind the severe hospital visiting rules in those early days. The pressure on her must have been huge.

The doctors felt there was nothing conclusive about Sheila's clinical state after this short period on a low phenylalanine diet, and Dr Bickel wrote (Bickel PhD, 1952):

'The assessment of any changes in mental capacity and behaviour of the patient presented great difficulties. The child was too young and of too low intelligence grade to be given any intelligence test. She behaved rather like a nine months old baby. There certainly was no sudden improvement under phenylalanine free food, apart for the fact that she soon became quieter and more contented and ceased banging her head on the pillow. This however might have been because she was now accustomed to her new environment. Livelier interest in her surroundings, a more intelligent expression in her eyes, attempts to stand, etc. were recorded by the nursing staff but are too vague to be indicative of any real improvement'.

Low Phenylalanine Diet at Home

Dr Hickmans: *'The diet is distasteful and monotonous'.*

The diet continued and after a four month period in hospital Sheila went home on 17th March 1952. Mary was to try the treatment for Sheila at home. The Birmingham team maintained the production of the special mixture in the laboratory and Mary would collect a supply each week, when Sheila would have weekly reviews of her condition with the doctors and regular blood tests. After a few weeks further modifications were made to the diet, with reductions in the amount of natural milk to only 100ml milk per day, as her blood phenylalanine level had risen too high. This severe restriction to her previous milk intake

7. Sheila's Treatment 1951-1953

required an increase in the amount of phenylalanine free hydrolysate to ensure Sheila was receiving enough protein equivalent. Sheila now had to drink 200ml of the unpleasant formula every day.

Initially the carbohydrate source was oatmeal or rice but this was changed to gluten-free wheat flour (wheat starch), presumably to keep the natural protein intake from the carbohydrate source as low as possible. There was some fruit and vegetables allowed and added sugar to try to make things more palatable, but it was still a very unappetizing diet. Compare the daily diet sheet with what would be the food for a two year old with PKU today.

The daily diet sheet for Mary to follow was (Bickel et al 1954):

8 a.m.	Gluten-free wheat flour *ad lib.* in water. 100 ml of milk, sugar *ad lib.*
10.30 a.m.	100 ml of the 10% phenylalanine-free casein hydrolysate.
11.30 a.m.	Orange juice with sugar.
1.30 p.m.	6-8 oz. cabbage, turnips or swedes boiled in water. 1 oz. butter, 1-2 oz. grated apple or banana. Sugar *ad lib.*
4 p.m.	10-12 oz. grated or cooked apples with sugar. Multivitamine drops, "Protovite" brand Roche, 1 ml daily.
6 p.m.	100 ml of the 10% phenylalanine-free casein hydrolysate.

This would have been a very difficult time for Mary looking after her family at Matlock Road. The city was still struggling after the war with food rationing continuing until 1954.

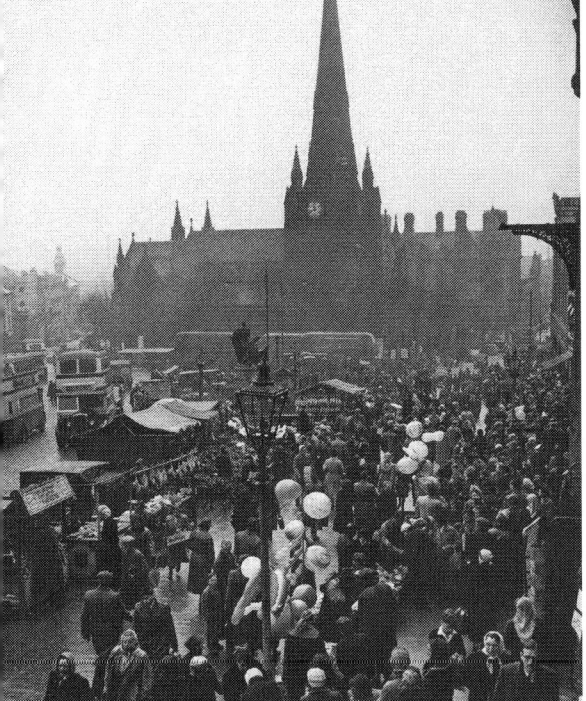

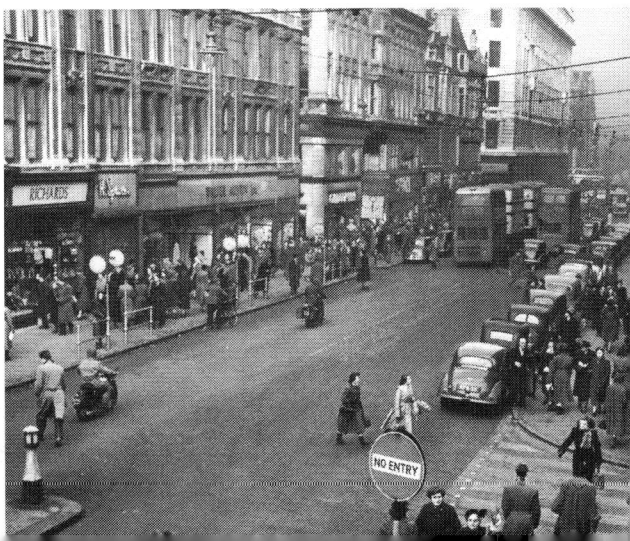

Left: Bullring market, Birmingham, 1950. Below: Corporation Street, Birmingham, December 1954 (photographs courtesy of Professor Carl Chinn).

There was little social care support in the community at this time and it would have been especially difficult as a single mother living at home with three small children, and no additional income other than from lodgers for a brief period. Mary would have to use the trams or buses for all her journeys. Living in Tyseley would have necessitated two journeys to get to the Children's Hospital, one into the city and then another bus to the hospital which was about two miles west from the city centre. Mary would make this journey every week with her severely handicapped two year old daughter in order to collect the 'mixture' for the following week and for the doctors to monitor Sheila's progress. On many of these weekly visits blood and urine samples would have been collected from Sheila to check that the diet was still having an effect. This was a huge undertaking for Mary – she was determined her daughter should have this treatment. She was doing her utmost, although there were no guarantees.

Terry remembers these times especially during school holidays when he would go with their Mum and Sheila on the bus, or sometimes on the tram, for the visits to the hospital. Sheila was a big girl and quite a handful. He remembers sitting in the waiting room at the hospital whilst Mary went into the clinic room to see the doctors with Sheila. The boys must have wondered what was going on and why Sheila needed this special mixture from a dark brown bottle which she didn't like. Why did she not have normal food like they did? They remember Mum collecting the diet every week and recall this large, heavy, dark glass bottle – which when they were shown a 2.5 litre *'Winchester'* bottle they said *'yes that was it!'*

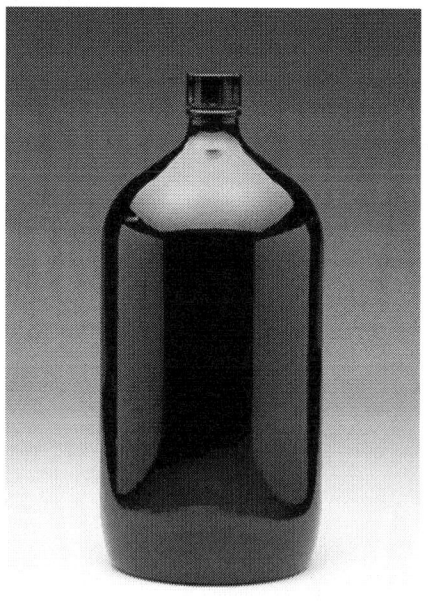

Winchester bottle for Sheila's Special Mixture.

A Winchester bottle is a clear or very dark brown (as in this case) thick glass laboratory bottle, very heavy when full, which is used in laboratories to store acids and solvents. The 2.5 litre bottle would have contained enough of the charcoal treated casein hydrolysate solution for a week's diet for Sheila.

Dr Hickmans (Appendix IV, set 1): *'the child was sent home on this carefully calculated diet sheet – the mother hugging a Winchester full of "the medicine" as well as carrying this rather heavy and awkward little girl'*. By now Sheila would have been nearly three years old.

7. Sheila's Treatment 1951-1953

It was very difficult to give Sheila this hugely unpleasant tasting formula with the rest of her diet being very restricted to small amounts of natural food. This would have been an enormous effort for Mary to keep this going every day; Terry and Trevor recall how Sheila struggled when given the bitter tasting acid mix, *'it looked like cold tea'*. It must have taken a lot of Mary's time to give Sheila her diet every day, watching over her to ensure she had all of the special mix and just as importantly nothing extra. Mary showed not only great determination in what she was doing but also courage to give her child this unproven and unpleasant product in the face of such practical difficulties and clear protestations from Sheila that she didn't want it. She must have had huge belief in what the doctors were doing for Sheila and hopeful of the benefits for her. Dr Bickel writes: *'the mother was very cooperative'* and reported that *'for months she adhered to the prescribed medicine'*.

At this stage the doctors began to note that there was a marked improvement in Sheila's demeanour when she came to the clinic over the next six months, especially in awareness and motor activity. Her eyes became brighter, she took more interest in her surroundings and in her food. She learnt to crawl, to stand, to push chairs and to climb up on to them. Her hair became thicker, began to shine and to change from a fair blonde colour to a dark brown colour. Roughness and eczema of the skin disappeared as did the musty mouse-like smell. All this happened whilst being on the diet at home over several months. The general impression from Mary Jones, and her neighbours was that there was a definite improvement.

The following was recorded in Dr Bickel's PhD thesis: *'Since Sheila returned home from hospital her eyes seem brighter and livelier than before. She plays more with toys, crawls more and tried to pull herself up. She makes noises as if she wants to talk. She begins to notice when her name is called whereas before she seemed deaf. She is interested in all food, crawls to pick up a biscuit from the floor and puts it into her mouth. This is the first time she has done this. She has nearly stopped rolling her head from side to side. She has now begun to quarrel with another baby about toys'*.

Although playing with other children was not part of Sheila's early life, and she did not go to nursery, this last statement confirms that she did have some interactions with others at this time. Trevor recalls a period when she was a *'bit better'* and there was another infant around – presumably someone for Sheila to play with.

It was not only the doctors who noted an improvement in Sheila's condition but also her mother. Mary reported to them that Sheila was livelier, played more and had more interest in her surroundings. By now it was October 1952 and Sheila was three years old and had been on the diet for 10 months. There was no doubt in the opinion of both the doctors and Mary that Sheila was benefitting from the special diet.

In the scientific publications that followed the changes were recorded with more detail. The darkening of Sheila's hair was explained by the addition of tyrosine to the diet. In PKU tyrosine, a precursor of the pigment melanin, is deficient because of the enzyme block and so the hair is abnormally fair in colour. Giving tyrosine enables melanin to be produced. Sheila now had eye contact, she smiled and stopped drooling and became more interested in her surroundings. Mary was convinced of progress but of course no one knew what would have happened if Sheila had not had the diet – would she have made these improvements anyway – maybe they were a result of the attention she was getting? The doctors could not be certain if this 10 month period of dietary treatment had been responsible for the changes they saw in Sheila or whether this was her development which would have happened anyway without the special diet.

The doctors were understandably questioning themselves about the quality of evidence they had. Some colleagues were expressing their scepticism about the findings as it is very difficult to scientifically evaluate developmental progress in such a young child over a short time frame. How could they be certain if it was the diet that was having an effect? It was critical to prove otherwise they would be no further forward in demonstrating that a low phenylalanine diet was of benefit in treating PKU. They also didn't know whether there would be any detrimental consequences from the diet, for example on Sheila's growth and other functions, especially longer term. Were they possibly introducing some as yet unknown problems for the future? The dilemma was also whether Sheila could continue on the diet. It was already very difficult to maintain the required intake of the special mix and would become more difficult as Sheila grew and would require more of the formula. Could it be justified to keep a young child on such an unpalatable diet? If they continued, how would this affect Sheila longer term? Would it be of benefit? Would there be harm? How long would they need to continue for? The dilemma was what to do? One can imagine the discussions.

The other critical question was the sheer practicalities of whether they could continue to make sufficient quantities of the homemade diet mixture in the laboratory. It was a very time consuming process with unrelenting pressure to keep up the production – a huge commitment for Horst Bickel and Evelyn Hickmans, knowing that this little girl was dependent on their preparation of the formula for her food. How much longer could they continue to produce the mixture in the laboratory, especially as increasing quantities were being required as Sheila grew? Dr Bickel was working day and night as evidenced by his family.

7. Sheila's Treatment 1951-1953

It was 1952 when his 16 year old niece from Germany came to live with the family in Solihull. She recalls:

'Already in those days we usually had our meals without Horst, as he was at the hospital during the day and often even at night. As soon as he arrived home, he would go to his favourite place, a wide couch, wrap a checked red rug around his legs and read medical journals and books. In the mornings he took me to school. I remember some conversations with him well: he tried to tell me how important it is to remain critical in all situations of life, towards people and also with regard to literature'.*

This last statement is particularly relevant in the events which followed.

*source – personal communication Bickel family 2019.

Phenylalanine Challenge

The next stage was a very bold step and one which by today's ethical standards could not have happened in this way. It reflected acceptable practice at the time and with hindsight was a critical stage in the history of PKU treatment. Without this step it would almost certainly have taken the Birmingham team longer to convince their medical and scientific colleagues of the benefits of dietary treatment, and the timeline for establishing newborn screening and treatment for PKU was likely to have been far longer.

The team decided to introduce a greater quantity of phenylalanine into Sheila's diet to mimic the amount she would be receiving on a normal diet and observe what happened i.e. to put Sheila back on a 'normal' diet in terms of phenylalanine content. They felt that only if this caused a deterioration in Sheila's condition could continuation of the phenylalanine low diet be justified. We assume from the records that there was no attempt to discuss this plan with Mary Jones at this point. They undertook this next stage of a phenylalanine challenge without Sheila's mother knowing – this was deliberate in order not to introduce a bias which might influence Mary's opinion.

The plan was to add 5g of pure l-phenylalanine to each day's supply of the phenylalanine free casein hydrolysate (special mixture) to mimic what Sheila would consume if receiving a normal diet. This commenced on 9th October 1952. Mary collected Sheila's weekly supply of the 'mix' in the Winchester bottle as normal but returned to the hospital some days later in tears and for the first time came without Sheila. She said that Sheila had lost in a few days all the ground she had gained whilst being on the diet and was back to the state she had been in prior to starting the diet almost a year earlier. Dr Bickel describes how they then visited Sheila's home at Matlock Road, six days after the extra phenylalanine had been introduced, to find Mary querying that a mistake must have been made with the diet. Why was Sheila like this? The two lodgers who knew the family well also commented that Sheila's condition had changed dramatically over the preceding week. She was not herself.

Dr Bickel and colleagues reported what Mary Jones had told them: *'Sheila within six hours of starting her "food" began to cry and roll and bang her head as she used to before being given the special diet. On the following day she had cried continually, her eyes had become heavy and she could no longer stand and scarcely crawl'*. These were dramatic descriptions of changes in Sheila's condition which had started immediately after the extra phenylalanine had been added. Mary was afraid that a mistake had been made with the mixture and therefore she had discontinued the *'food'*, and within a few days Sheila had begun to recover. After the doctors' visit, Sheila was promptly put back on the phenylalanine reduced diet and very soon, another six days later, she was back to how she had been before this change. The doctors saw Sheila again on 23rd October when she seemed back to her normal self, prior to this challenge.

We don't know how Mrs Jones reacted to what the doctors then told her i.e. that Sheila had been deliberately given a mixture with added phenylalanine so they could find out what would happen. We can only assume that she understood the reasoning as the doctors then asked for her consent to repeat the challenge, but this time in hospital under observation with laboratory investigations and moreover to film Sheila. The doctors felt that this reaction to the extra phenylalanine in her diet was so important to confirm, that they needed to repeat it. Mary agreed to this so we can only deduce that she appreciated the huge importance of doing it to produce the evidence that the doctors needed to report their findings and to help others. She would have known that it would cause Sheila further distress, not to mention how upsetting it would be to herself and for Sheila to have to go back into hospital. This could not have been an easy decision and shows a level of understanding of the importance and trust in what the doctors were trying to do. It would have been easier and perhaps more understandable if Mary had insisted that Sheila continue on the phenylalanine reduced diet as clearly, Mary herself was convinced of the benefits for her daughter. Agreement to repeat the challenge was done for the potential benefits of others. We can only imagine how it must have felt to see her daughter becoming so unwell, unhappy and upset and then agreeing to do it all again. She had great confidence in the Birmingham team and moreover understood the implications for others with PKU for the future. Mary's courage and selflessness cannot be understated.

7. Sheila's Treatment 1951-1953

Third Admission to BCH – Challenge Repeated

In order to confirm Mary Jones' observations Sheila was admitted for the third time to BCH on 5th November 1952 whilst established back on the low phenylalanine diet. She was observed for a period of time and as a record of these events filming was undertaken by Dr Bickel. The following photographs are taken from this film (BCH Archive; compilation of films 2008) with special thanks to Tom Chimiak, film maker (photographs reproduced with kind permission of the Jones Family). Sheila was alert, playing and interested although still obviously mentally impaired; she walked with support and laughed when tickled. In the film Dr Bickel uses his keys to get Sheila's attention and play with.

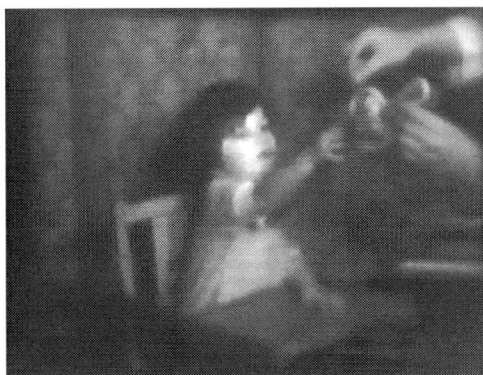 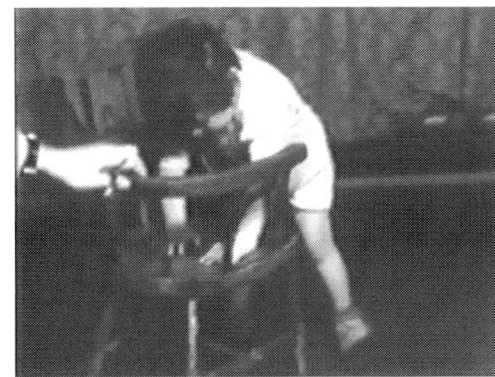

Sheila 11 months after starting phenylalanine restricted diet.

Three weeks later on 26th November 4g l- phenylalanine was added to her diet and the following day, 5g added. The changes in her behaviour were impressive and dramatic with a very disturbed noisy night unlike the other nights spent in hospital. She had to be sedated. Within 24 hours she became increasingly irritable, drowsy and vomited; her facial expressions, particularly her eyes became vacant and she lost interest in her food and surroundings. She developed facial eczema and began to salivate. After 6 days with the added phenylalanine she could no longer stand or crawl and was not interested in toys or Dr Bickel's keys.

On 3rd December the additional phenylalanine was discontinued and she was put back on the phenylalanine reduced diet. Some weeks later Sheila was able to walk again with support of a chair. She was a lot more interested in playing, with a little smile, and able to crawl onto and under a chair.

These remarkable and highly important findings were published initially as a preliminary communication (Bickel et al 1953). This was the first time that a person with phenylketonuria had been given a diet low in phenylalanine. Full details with

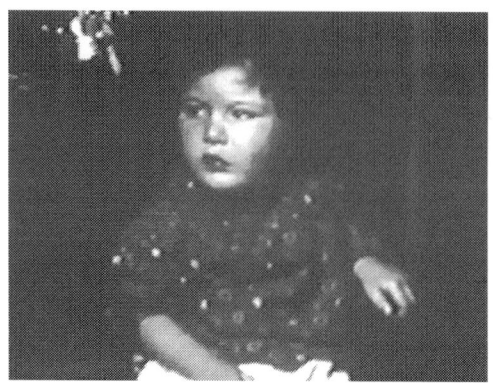 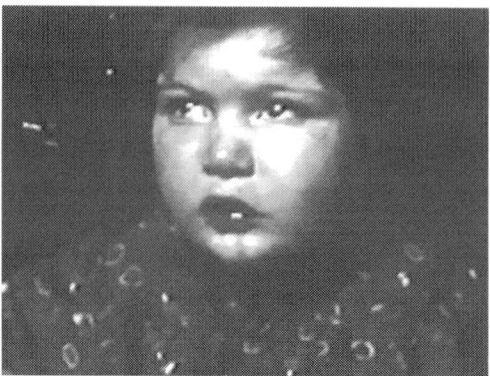

Sheila with phenylalanine added to her diet.

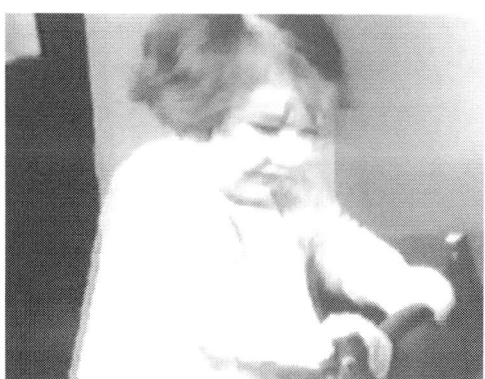 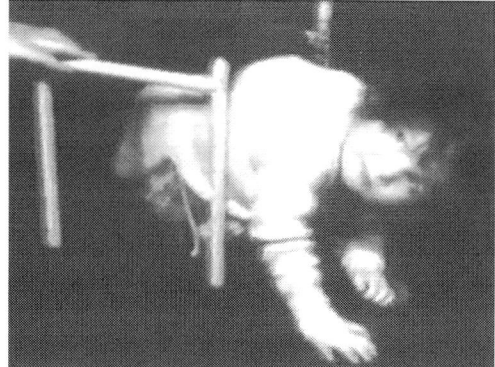

Sheila one year after starting phenylalanine restricted diet.

results of the biochemical investigations documenting the changes in Sheila's blood and urine phenylalanine were subsequently reported (see opposite).

The authors concluded that their findings clearly suggest that excess phenylalanine or its breakdown products have a deleterious action on mental function in PKU. An important question raised at the time was what would happen if phenylalanine was given to non PKU individuals? Would there be a similar adverse effect? Although previous work giving a single dose of phenylalanine to non PKU subjects showed no observed deleterious effects, Dr Bickel subsequently gave a five month old child without PKU four grams l-phenylalanine for four days. There was no untoward reaction (Bickel 1954), albeit the extent of the rise in blood phenylalanine was significantly lower (x15) in the normal child than that observed in PKU. So although not directly comparable these findings suggested the deleterious effect of added dietary

7. Sheila's Treatment 1951-1953

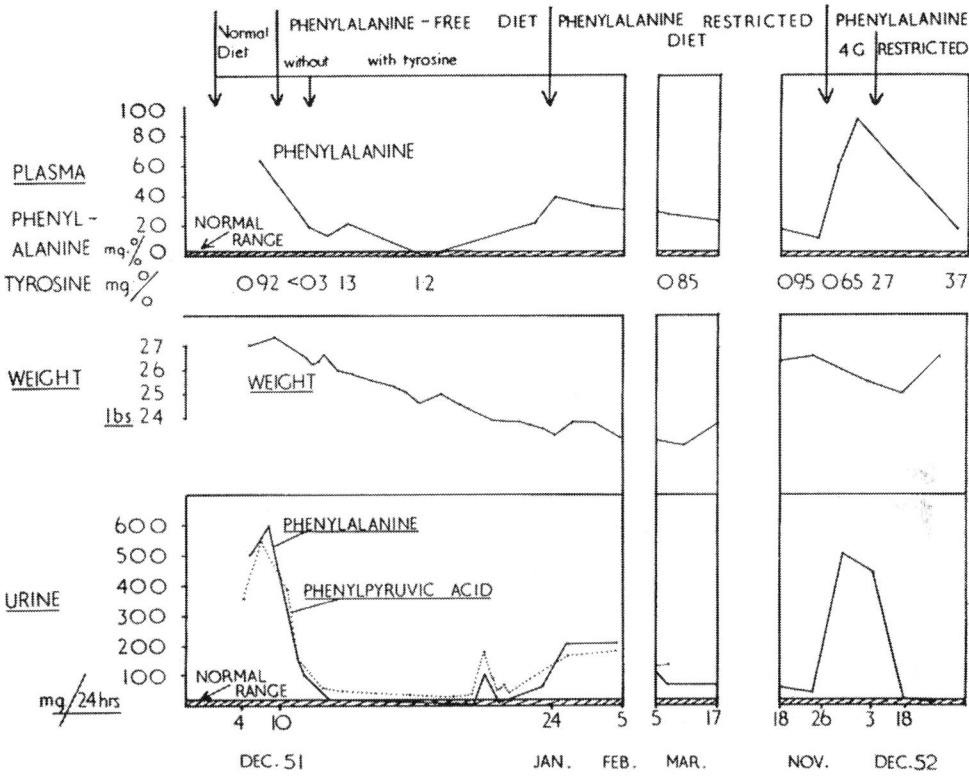

The influence of a phenylalanine free and a phenylalanine restricted diet on Sheila's biochemistry and her body weight (reproduced from Bickel, H. et al 1954).

phenylalanine was specific to PKU and reflects the susceptibility of the brain in the condition. The authors also concluded that the aim of treatment with a low phenylalanine diet is to keep the phenylalanine blood level near normal without going into negative nitrogen balance, as initially had occurred with Sheila when the phenylalanine free product was given and she lost weight. The importance of checking the response to a diet by measuring phenylalanine in blood was recognised and stimulated the development of better methods for analysis.

The Birmingham team concluded that the value of using such a diet for treatment of PKU could only be truly assessed by further trials with more patients, but that it would be unlikely to benefit older children already with mental deficiency because permanent damage would probably already have occurred. It was correctly assumed at that early stage that the best results will be obtained if treatment is started in early infancy, particularly in the neonatal period, a conclusion which is now well established and is the basis for the newborn screening programmes for PKU across the world.

1953 – What Next?

After the publication of Sheila's dietary trial further developments then occurred very quickly. There was initially scepticism from some quarters with suggestions that the findings from Birmingham were far too speculative on which to base recommendations for treatment. It was therefore very important to try the treatment on more cases and document any changes in the development of each individual. Others around the world were now encouraged to attempt dietary treatment for PKU and to provide further evidence. Independently, work in the USA (Armstrong and Tyler 1955) reported treatment of five PKU cases with a low phenylalanine diet comprising a mixture of pure l-amino acids as 'protein substitute' as opposed to a casein hydrolysate source. Less conclusive evidence of the potential clinical benefits was obtained although the biochemistry was normalised.

Louis Woolf, at Great Ormond Street Hospital in London, galvanised by the findings from Sheila, soon repeated the work (Woolf 1955) in two children both aged 2 years, 8 months and an older child 5 years, 5 months (two idiots and one imbecile) but this time with more objective psychometric and EEG measurements. The children were fed, like Sheila, a diet of phenylalanine low casein hydrolysate as the protein source, except that it was now commercially available as a dry powder. The diet was given for nine and ten months respectively in the two younger children and four months in the older child. Marked intellectual improvement resulted in the two younger children and in one case the EEG became normal; interestingly in all cases their hair, originally very pale, became darker during the treatment. The results of the psychological testing showed that there was considerable intellectual improvement with increase in IQ and improvements in development.

During 1953 Sheila had continued to be treated with a low phenylalanine diet at home but it was around this time the team from BCH began to go their separate ways. Dr Hickmans retired in 1953, Dr Bickel, after gaining his PhD, returned to Germany in 1954 and in 1955 Dr Gerrard left BCH to become head of Paediatrics in Saskatchewan, Canada. The value of the diet was still being questioned and more cases needed to be studied.

8

SHEILA 1953-1956

Professor Gerrard reflected in 1987: 'if only we had known that we were helping her (Sheila) more than we understood we might have insisted that someone at least kept an eye on her when we left'.

Further Cases at Birmingham

Sheila and by now several other infants with PKU were simultaneously being treated in Birmingham. These patients were under the care of various consultant Paediatricians at BCH – Dr Gerrard (until 1955), Dr Otto Wolff and Professor Smellie. The Birmingham doctors who continued the work of Dr Bickel and Dr Gerrard had now been treating six PKU patients with diet, not just Sheila.

There was an acknowledgment in the 1953 publication from Birmingham that the phenylalanine 'free' casein hydrolysate, initially prepared in the laboratory, had begun to be obtained commercially. The formula as a low phenylalanine protein substitute was now being obtained from Allen and Hanburys. This was a very rapid response from industry – a clear recognition of the huge importance of the findings from BCH and the potential need for such a product.

The specialised laboratory testing required to monitor treatment was now an order of magnitude greater, with several patients simultaneously on the diet. Evelyn Hickmans had retired and laboratory work was now being undertaken by Drs Blainey and Gulliford, from the University of Birmingham, at the metabolic research unit at Little Bromwich Hospital, Birmingham (this subsequently became East Birmingham Hospital and is now Heartlands Hospital). It was formerly a hospital for infectious diseases and had only become a General Hospital in 1953. In 1956 findings from six cases (including Sheila) in whom detailed metabolic studies and formal testing of IQ and development had been undertaken were reported (Blainey and Gulliford 1956). Improvements in mental age and IQ were shown in these cases. All these results added to the strength of evidence which was emerging of the value of a low phenylalanine diet for treating PKU.

Sheila, after the period on the diet from December 1951 to October 1952 and the phenylalanine challenge in late 1952, had remained at home on the diet with continuation of the frequent hospital outpatient visits. It is not clear if all of the follow up visits were at the Children's Hospital as reference is made to attending outpatients at Little Bromwich Hospital. Little Bromwich (ref Map Birmingham, 7) was closer to Sheila's home in Tyseley at the time and this was maybe a reason why the follow up location changed from the Children's Hospital.

Developmental Assessments
When treatment for Sheila was first started in December 1951 her development was not assessed formally; such testing was not well established as a tool within Paediatrics at that time. Several techniques to evaluate the mental ability in this young age group were being developed but it was only in 1953 that they became part of Sheila's evaluation. Although we don't have continuous detailed records on Sheila to refer to, the periodic assessments of her mental progress and those of five other children with PKU in Birmingham, who were all being given a phenylalanine reduced diet, were reported (Blainey and Gulliford 1956). These assessments of the mental progress of Sheila are summarised below.

To recap, in December 1952 after one year on the diet she was able to walk with the support of a chair, was interested in playing and able to crawl onto a chair. Now at the commencement of more formal developmental testing aged 3 years 7 months, after 17 months of phenylalanine restriction, Sheila could stand with the aid of furniture, would climb on a chair, crawl actively and explore cupboards and objects at floor level. She was indifferent to toys unless they made a noise or moved e.g. a ball or spinning top. She could not hold two objects at once but the thumb was beginning to be used in manipulation. She made some two syllable babble and kissing noises. Her attention span was limited and she quickly tired, cried and would lay rocking on the floor. Her mental age was assessed as 10 months. There was an improvement in many features, except speech, in this first year of receiving the diet.

After two years of treatment in January 1954 (aged 4 years 3 months) she was now able to stand unaided and could walk a few steps with help. Her attention span was markedly increased and she was interested in more objects; thumb opposition was complete and she could pick up a pellet neatly and place one brick on another. She could make a stroke with a pencil and looked briefly at a picture book. Apart from language, which continued to lag markedly, she was assessed overall as at about the 12 months level.

In May 1954, 12 months after the first assessment and 2 years and 5 months after the start of treatment, she was now walking alone, able to climb into a child's push-along wagon and could sit in a small chair. She was a lot more interested in playing and particularly more interested in playing with toys, trying to spin a top by pumping the handle and building a tower with cubes. She would

8. Sheila 1953-1956

fill a cup with cubes, scribble with a pencil and look at a picture book. Apart from speech, which still hadn't progressed, she had gained five months of mental development in this 12 month period. Motor development was rated at 18 months and in other aspects she was at 15 months.

In 1954 there was further film evidence from BCH showing her improvements. She was filmed sat on her Mum's lap building a brick tower, looking at a picture book and was generally able to respond to people. It was assessed that she had gained around six to seven months in development during the period of being on a phenylalanine reduced diet. The last section of the film we have is in the winter of 1954 with Sheila walking on her own down a snow covered path in front of the laboratory block at BCH (BCH Archive; compilation of films 2008).

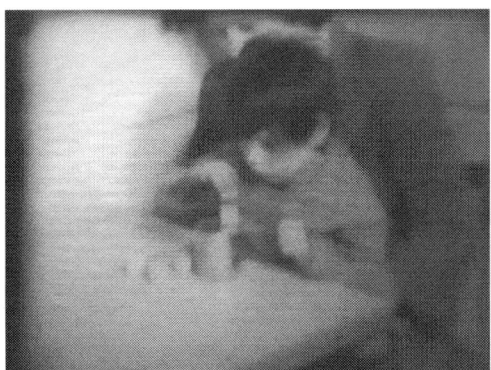
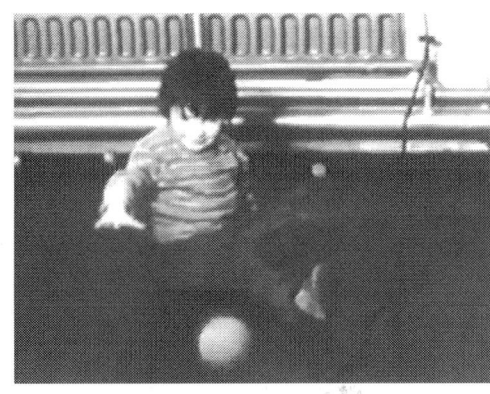

Sheila on her Mum's lap building a brick tower and playing with a ball.

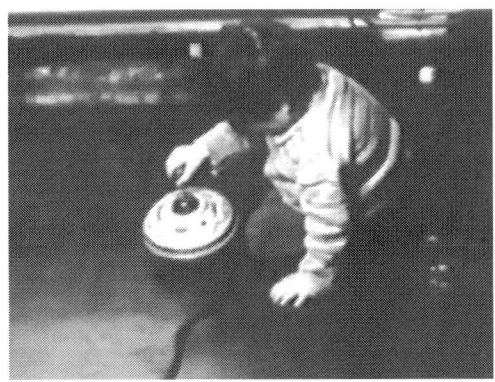
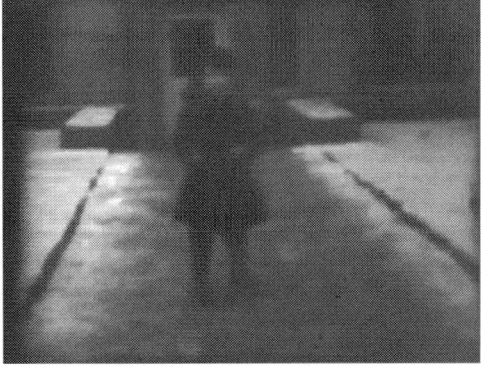

Sheila playing with a top and walking in front of laboratory block at BCH (photographs reproduced with kind permission of the Jones Family).

In February 1955, at 5 years 4 months, Sheila was assessed for the first time using the Griffiths scale. This was a new method of assessment developed in 1954 by Ruth Griffiths, a psychologist whose observations of children from birth to eight years in age over six areas enabled a measure of development as a complete profile of skills. This was a unique approach and a huge advance in assessing how an individual young infant was progressing over time. Using this scale showed that Sheila's motor development had further improved and she could walk kicking a ball and could squat in play. She again made a tower of bricks, scribbled with a pencil and liked to carry a doll. She drank from a cup and was able to point to indicate her needs. Language continued to lag. Overall progress had continued but at a slower rate than the preceding 12 months. There was considerable variation in the different aspects of her development as indicated by the results of this first testing using the Griffiths scale. Of particular note was her continued lack of language.

Deteriorating Dietary Control
In November 1954 Mary Jones had a fourth child, Philip, and this coincided with worsening of Sheila's dietary control. Her plasma phenylalanine levels increased, her urine contained excess phenylalanine and the ferric chloride test became positive. During this period there was considerable gain in her weight which had been stationary for much of the period 1953-1955. All these findings (see opposite) suggested that Mary was no longer able to manage for Sheila to stay on her diet. This was at variance from the early days of treatment and an indication that all was not well. There had been a deterioration in home circumstances associated with this poor dietary control. The family were still at Matlock Road but now Mary had a baby and two young boys as well as Sheila to look after. Trevor and Terry, after a period at a nursery, were now at the local junior school at Yarnfield Road, Tyseley. The boys went to and from school on their own and had little help from Mary who was doing her utmost to cope with the increasing demands of looking after Sheila, now five years old, and a new baby.

Attempts to keep Sheila's dietary phenylalanine restricted using the low phenylalanine mixture continued until November 1955. At that point, in view of the clear difficulties in her continuing with the special mixture, efforts were relaxed and in December 1955 the phenylalanine low casein hydrolysate mixture was discontinued. Phenylalanine intake was limited with a low intake of natural protein. In December 1955 at 6 years 2 months the poor dietary control was reflected in Sheila's manner. She was more easily distracted and test materials for the developmental assessments were thrown on the floor. Nevertheless some further progress was recorded, she could now use a cup and spoon by herself and could

8. Sheila 1953-1956

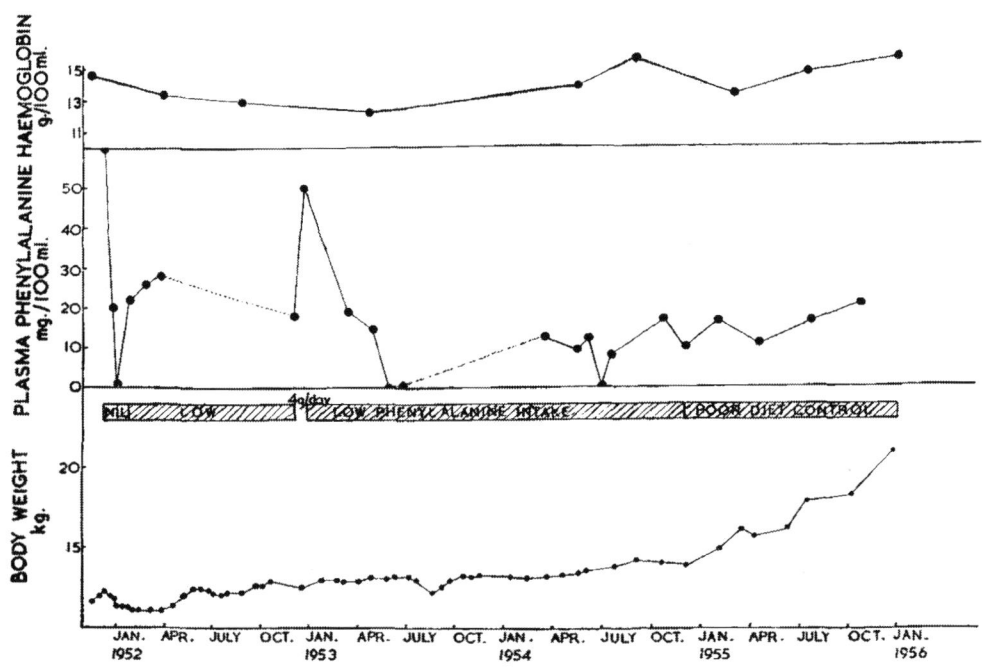

Changes in plasma phenylalanine and body weight for Sheila 1952-1956 (reproduced from Blainey, J.D. and Gulliford, R., 1956).

take the wrapping paper off a sweet, and would walk along pulling a toy. After being on a low protein diet for the next five months Mary claimed Sheila was well and had continued to acquire new activities at home. However, the doctors found Sheila to be uncooperative and distracted and, when developmental testing was attempted, her mental ability was judged to have progressed at a considerably lower rate than previously. The assessment in April 1956, when she was 6 years and 6 months, is the last record we have during Sheila's childhood. She was not adhering to the low protein diet very well and making little progress; she was judged to be functioning at a mental age of around 18 months. This was clearly very disappointing in view of her earlier progress. Why did things go wrong at this stage?

It is understandable that with the three key figures having left BCH, and more PKU cases now being treated, that the medical focus on Sheila would be much less. The other professionals in Birmingham who had continued with the work, had turned their attention to treatment for newly diagnosed cases at a younger age and the establishment of screening programmes. The last information we have is a reference by Dr Gerrard to a letter from Dr Blainey to her family doctor Dr Allin on 28th July 1955 about Sheila's progress (Dr Gerrard – clinical notes). Further clinical records from BCH have not been found suggesting it was the end of her follow up there.

1956 also coincided with the family moving home from Matlock Road to Aston, a poor deprived area just north of the city centre (ref Map Birmingham, 8). It is unclear why the family made this move other than perhaps financial hardship prevented the family from staying at Matlock Road. The demands on Mary of looking after Sheila were enormous as she now had four children to look after, including a young baby. She had her boys to care for and it had just become too difficult to continue with Sheila's diet.

The move of the family across to the north of the city in 1956 would seem to coincide with the end of Sheila's detailed follow up by the doctors, either at BCH or Little Bromwich Hospital. The NHS, still in its early years, was not systematic in follow up and the hospitals were not joined up with the community services. Computerised records were decades away and there would be no process to ensure Sheila's follow up. PKU was a relatively new disorder and rare. The professionals involved in community care at the time would be battling with much bigger issues of poverty, malnutrition and infectious diseases. PKU would be 'small print'.

There would have been no one supporting Mary to help her cope with the diet as Sheila was getting older. She was now almost seven years old but with the skills of a two year old or less and there was no one to help with the family or home. The burden facing Mary must have been huge and she was understandably under great stress. She must have had big questions in her mind about the future for Sheila. Would she ever be able to speak? Would she ever be able to look after herself? It is understandable that Mary found it all too much to maintain Sheila's diet in the context of her family circumstances and perhaps no longer held any real hope that Sheila would get better. It was the end of the diet for Sheila.

After 1956 nothing further was published about Sheila's treatment and there are no hospital records of Sheila's care from 1956 until her subsequent admission to Chelmsley Hospital in 1959 (see p.66). Horst Bickel felt a great sadness that no one in the medical services knew what had happened to Sheila after this time. There were unsubstantiated stories that *'Mrs Jones was no longer able to continue the diet and had abandoned it'*. As a statement this may be true but does not take into account the personal and family circumstances Mary was facing. She was on her own providing constant care and attention for Sheila, by now a strong seven year old, and not knowing what the future might look like for her daughter.

9

THE FAMILY STORY – PART II: THE 'LOST YEARS' 1956-1959

Trevor Jones: 'A disaster. We went from a nice maisonette, with a lounge, two bedrooms, a bathroom, hot and cold water and we went to a back house – we called it a back yard'.

Life at Victoria Road, Aston

It was in 1956 that the family had moved from Matlock Road to Victoria Road, Aston to live in a back-to-back house (see Appendix I; Carl Chinn 2013). Aston was a very deprived working class area of inner city Birmingham, with streets of old red brick Victorian houses. The area still showed the effects of bomb damage from the war with areas of derelict land and partly demolished houses. Much of the housing in the area was subsequently demolished in the late 1960s to make way for the Aston Expressway, a multi-lane link for transport from the national motorway network to the city centre which opened in 1972.

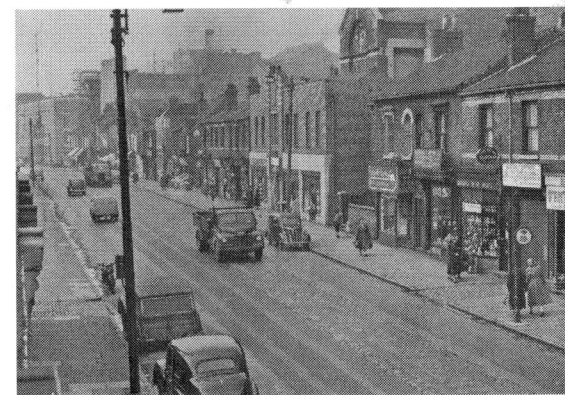

Lichfield Road looking towards Victoria Road, Aston (photograph courtesy of Professor Carl Chinn).

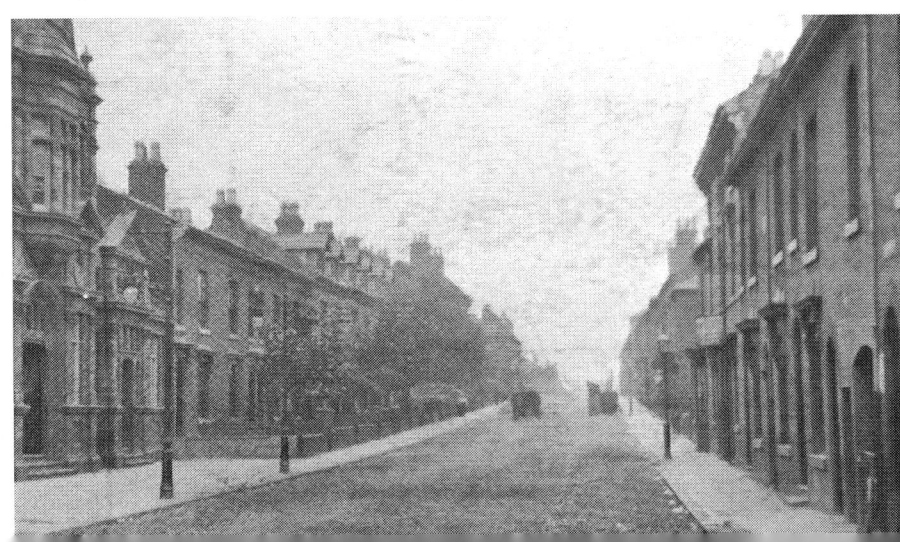

Victoria Road (photograph courtesy of Birmingham Libraries).

A personal anecdote from the author:

'When I started work in 1968 at the old General hospital on Steelhouse Lane (now the Children's Hospital) before the Aston Expressway was completed I drove "nose to tail" on the old A38 road through this area of Aston on a daily basis. The air was full of exhaust fumes and the strong overpowering spice smells from the nearby HP sauce factory. One of my earliest memories of Birmingham was acid rain falling on my nylon stockings which instantaneously disintegrated into huge red-edged holes. Keeping the car windows closed was essential!'

The back-to-back house in which the Jones family lived was typical of much of the housing of that era in inner city Birmingham. These houses were built as rows of terraces facing onto the street with another row joined to their back walls, with a single brick in between. Those at the back faced into a shared inner courtyard, usually referred to as the yard. Each house had a single door which opened from the living room either directly onto the street or the inner yard. To get from the street to the shared inner yard was via a narrow entry or gap between two houses. The houses were very small with cramped conditions, typically three storeys with a small kitchen, one bedroom, one living room, an attic and a cellar. The living room also served as a dining room, work room for jobs, drying washing if it was a wet day and much more. The houses were dark and poorly ventilated with only one door to the outside. There was on open area in the yard for rubbish and a communal wash house. By the 1950s most had a cold water supply to the house. The shared wash house had a coal-fired copper boiler used

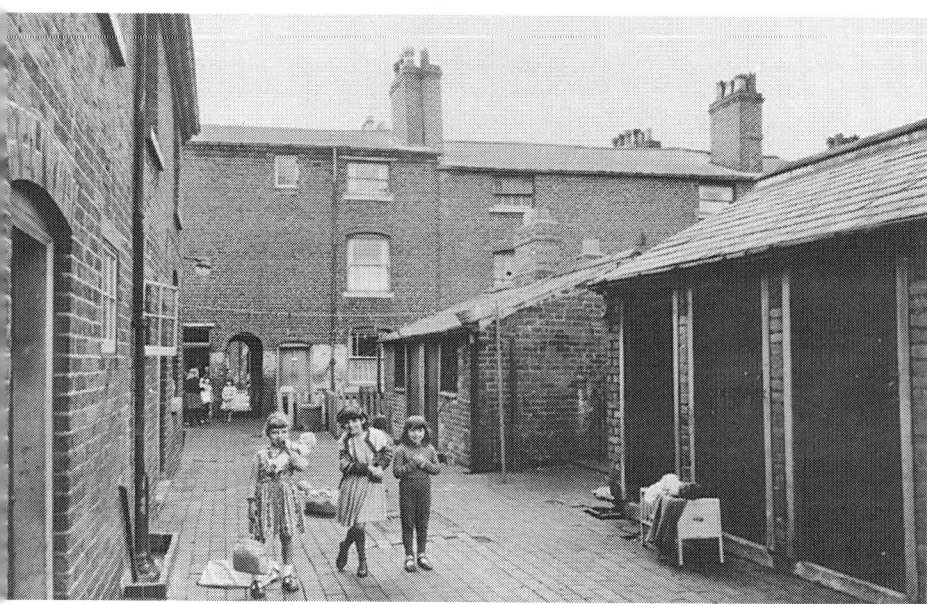

Back-to-Back Houses, Birmingham, early 1960s (photograph courtesy of Professor Carl Chinn).

9. The Family Story – Part II

to heat the water for wash days. Outside lavatories, in the yard, were shared between several families. The yard was where the children played and the washing hung out to dry. There were usually no gardens.

Most of this back-to-back housing has since been demolished across the city although there is a small renovated area close to the city centre, albeit not at Aston, which is now a museum (National Trust). A visit gives some appreciation of the conditions which families faced but living in one of these back-to-backs can only really be understood by those who actually lived there.

Where the Jones family lived there were about 30 of these 'back' houses grouped together with an archway from the road into the shared courtyard and a path to the single door of number 14 – back of 193, Victoria Road.

Sheila's brothers Terry and Trevor recall the move to Aston: *'I just don't know why we went there. It was a shock. Whoever got our house at Matlock Road must have been amazed about how nice it was. I think our Mum saw an advert in the paper for a house swap. At Aston we went through the door directly into a living area – just one room with lino on the floor. There was a settee and single chair, a cabinet with the radio and a small cupboard with the black and white TV – oh yes and a large table which always had lots of stuff on top. We had a tiny, tiny kitchen with a flagged stone floor which had a gas cooker and a sink with a cold water tap – there was no space for work surfaces. There was no hot water'.* Somehow Mary managed to prepare food in this kitchen for her family. *'From the living room there was a door leading to the steps down to the cellar – that's where we kept coal. Another door opened to the steep narrow staircase which led upstairs to the one bedroom and then from there another flight of narrow stairs to the attic. The only heating was an open coal fire in the living area – there was a tiled fireplace and a grate. We always had a fireguard and that's where Sheila would sit on her blanket in front of the fire. Washing was done in a separate communal building in the yard – we called it the Brew House (pronounced brewus) – on a Monday morning. Mum would dry clothes on a line in the yard. The only toilet was a long way from the house and shared with two other houses. In the house hot water had to be heated up in a kettle and we had a tin bath. I would have a 'strip' wash in the kitchen and then go to the local swimming baths on a Friday. There was four of us and Mum'.*

Mary didn't tell the boys anything about why they had moved but they think the reason was associated with Mary's deteriorating health. *'How the authorities agreed to the move I just don't know; it was not a nice time'.* The family had very little and the brothers remember it as an extremely difficult time living in such poor accommodation with little income for the family. Mary had an early morning cleaning job at a bank at Aston Cross. *'She used to get up early in a morning before we went to school'* – presumably leaving the children at home asleep. Initially there was no support or help for Mary whilst she continued her struggle to care for Sheila at home and little or no help for herself to deal with the increasing stress she was under. In those days there would have been a stigma associated with having a child who was referred to as mentally retarded. It was the very early days for any help from Social Services, and PKU would not be known about to the case workers who subsequently had contact with the family.

Mary continued to look after her family in these conditions for a further two years but in 1958 she had what her sons describe as 'a nervous breakdown' and sought help. She was admitted in September 1958 and again in March 1959 to a local Psychiatric unit (Highcroft Hospital), usually referred to as the asylum, for short term care; in both cases this was on a voluntary basis for a period of three weeks and 16 weeks respectively.

Mary at Highcroft Hospital

Dr Hickmans: *'Sheila's mother had succumbed to all her worries looking after her children for so long and is now in a mental hospital suffering from a complete mental breakdown'.*

Highcroft Hospital, founded 1836, was located just north of the City centre and not far from the Jones' family home at Aston, (see Map Birmingham, 9), it was formerly Aston Union Workhouse and Infirmary (see Appendices II and III). It was developed into a larger workhouse and infirmary and was subsequently named Erdington House in 1912. With the introduction of the NHS in 1948 the Victorian workhouse and infirmary buildings became Highcroft Hall Hospital (usually shortened to Highcroft Hospital) and used primarily as a psychiatric hospital caring for long term chronic and short term acute patients with mental and nervous disorders. It appears to have been also used as a maternity unit in the post WWII baby boom and this is where Trevor had been born in 1945. In 1979 there were 853 beds for the mentally ill. In 1996 it was closed for redevelopment like the other large mental institutions in Birmingham.

The archived records of Highcroft Hospital are limited but confirm that Mary was admitted in September 1958 for 3 weeks as a voluntary patient for psychiatric treatment. During this time Sheila was cared for in a mental deficiency hospital specifically for children (Chelmsley Hospital). Little is known about Mary's treatment at Highcroft other than she was sufficiently improved to be discharged after just a few weeks with her condition described as 'relieved'. However Mary was admitted for a second time to Highcroft, six months later in March 1959, and Sheila was again admitted to Chelmsley Hospital. Terry and Trevor remember being taken to Highcroft Hospital for visits to see their Mum. Asylums were very

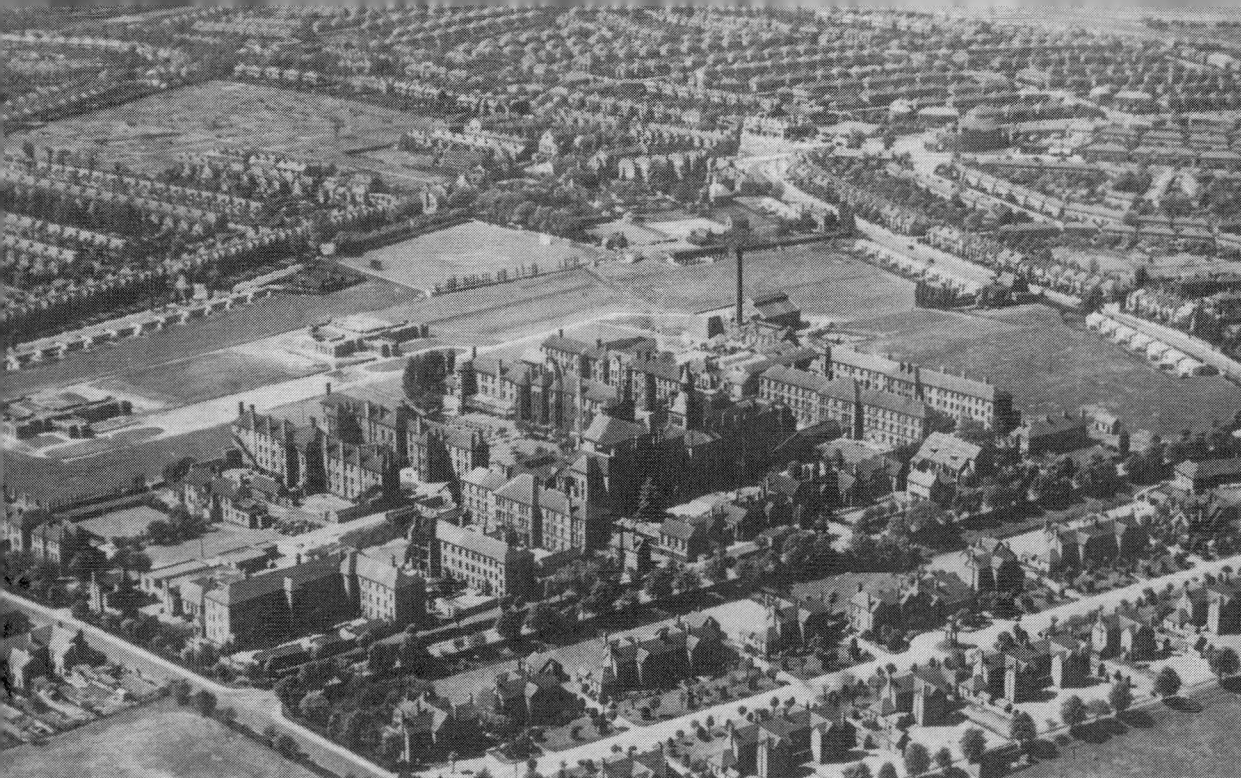

*Highcroft Hall Hospital, Erdington, Birmingham, c.1930s
(photograph copyright courtesy of Mary Evans / Peter Higginbotham Collection).*

frightening places so these were traumatic experiences for the young boys. Mary was pregnant at the time of her second admission and so she was transferred to St Chads, a maternity unit in Birmingham, close to the Children's Hospital for the birth of William (Liam) in June 1959.

During these two periods in 1958 and 1959 when Mary was in hospital Terry, Trevor and Philip were taken into care at two different local Children's homes – Shenley Cottage Homes at Shenley Fields (Northfield, Birmingham) and Father Hudson's in Coleshill – these were not happy experiences for the brothers.

'Mum was pregnant with Liam – Social Services came and took us to the Children's home – for about six weeks – it felt like six months.' Philip was only four years old. 'They took us in the back of a van. When we came home there was a pram in the living room with Liam. Sheila was not there when we came home'.

After returning home from her second admission to Highcroft, Mary was still under stress, having not yet regained her normal self. After three years living in the back yard house at Aston and now looking after her five children including a baby of four weeks, this was the tipping point for Mary with the realisation that she could no longer look after Sheila at home. In July 1959 whilst at home, and when the three older boys were on 'holiday leave' at Shenley Cottage Homes, Mary applied for Sheila to be admitted to a mental deficiency hospital – this was Chelmsley Hospital.

10

SHEILA AT CHELMSLEY HOSPITAL

Terry and Trevor Jones: *'Mum was not well'*.

Context and History of Chelmsley Hospital
The provision of services and care for individuals with learning disabilities who have mental health and behaviour problems has seen enormous changes during the timeline of this story. The stigma of learning disability led to a succession of changes in terminology which has happened in parallel with changes in the organisation of services over this period. Appendix III provides the reader with background information about Mental Health Services in the UK which sets the context for Sheila's care at Chelmsley.

It was 2nd September 1958 when Sheila was first admitted to Chelmsley Hospital (formerly Coleshill Hall Mental Hospital), near Coleshill, on the east side of Birmingham for short term care – this coincided with Mary's first admission to Highcroft Hospital. Sheila stayed at Chelmsley for about five weeks on this first occasion and was discharged on 7th October 1958. Sheila had a second admission on 21st February 1959 again to coincide with Mary's admission to Highcroft. We assume Sheila's care was organised on both occasions so Mary was able to obtain respite and treatment for herself.

These two short term admissions subsequently led Mary to arrange for Sheila's permanent admission to Chelmsley Hospital on 25th July 1959 as a 'mental defective'. Mary had requested that she be admitted under the legislation of the Mental Deficiency Act and Sheila was *'accepted as an informal patient at the request of the patient's mother'*. As this was a voluntary admission at Mary's request and under the legislation Sheila would not be under any specific restrictions.

Chelmsley Hospital, as part of the NHS, has a long history of caring for those individuals with mental deficiency and at the time of Sheila's admission was looking after mainly children. The hospital was originally built in 1878/9 as Marston Green Cottage Homes and was part of the workhouse system for Birmingham located on the east side of the city (see Map Birmingham, 10). Its original purpose was to provide accommodation out in the country for pauper children – these were orphans or poor children from the city who had no one to look after them. By 1904 it was

10. Sheila at Chelmsley Hospital

accommodating 420 children which rose to 510 in 1911. Further buildings were added in 1923. After 1930 the site became Coleshill Hall Mental Hospital caring for 'individuals who were deemed to be mental defectives' and was renamed Chelmsley Hospital around 1956. Chelmsley was initially for mentally defective children below the age of about 12 years and as young as two years.

The hospital had several large separate blocks containing the wards. It was a self-contained 'village' with a church, swimming pool, school, kitchen, laundry, leisure centre/recreation block, garden and in the early days a farm and workshop. At its peak capacity in the early 1970s there would be around 1000 patients segregated into male and female wards each housing on average 30-40 individuals, although sometimes many more especially in the earlier years. The patients were of varying abilities and classified into different categories according to the Mental Deficiency Act (see Appendix III) and as the children grew into adulthood the age range became extremely wide with one lady at the time of the hospital closure almost 100 years of age. Although there was a school on site, prior to the Education Act of 1970, there was no requirement for education to be provided so those children like Sheila with a severe learning disability would not receive any education. After 1970 children were no longer admitted to Chelmsley. However, children's wards remained for many years until all those admitted prior to 1970 had become adults. The hospital existed until 1999 when it was closed and the site was partly demolished for redevelopment as

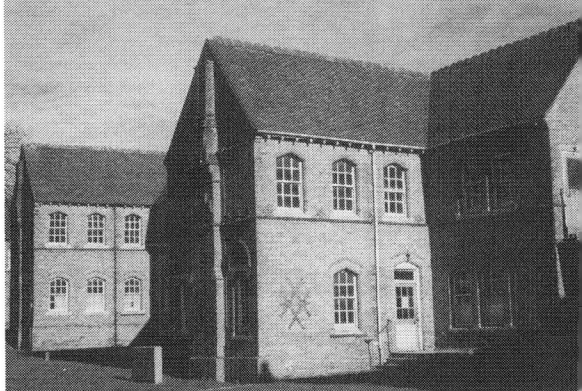

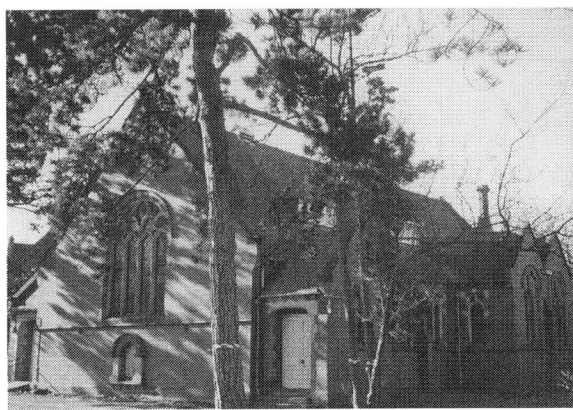

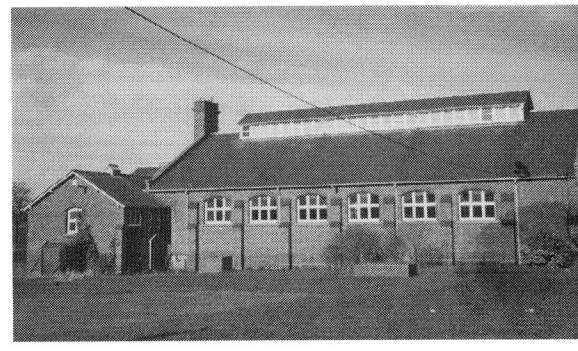

Chelmsley Hospital
Top: Ward Blocks; Middle: Church.
Bottom: Leisure Centre (Recreation Hall) (photographs kindly provided by Brooklands Hospital).

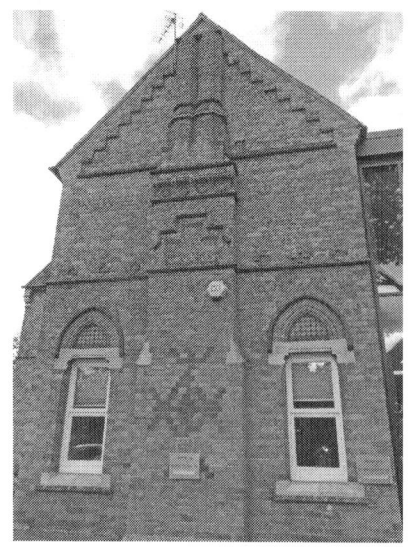
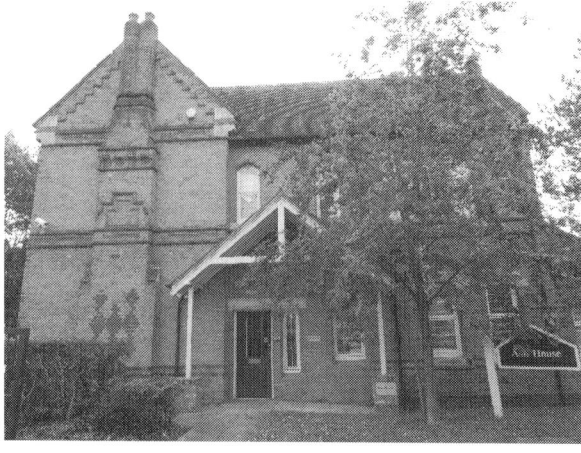

*Former Chelmsley Hospital buildings in 2019.
Above: Gatehouse. Left: Reception/offices.*

houses and offices/businesses. A few of the original buildings still exist in 2019 as part of the new business park development (see photographs above).

Admission 1959

Trevor: *'It is hard to believe that our Mum kept Sheila at home for so long with no help. When I think about what help she would get today and what would be available, I feel sad'.*

It must have been agonising for Mary to see Sheila effectively taken into care into a large asylum (although at her request) after all she had fought for and done for her only daughter. She had been so determined to get treatment and for over four years had been backwards and forwards to the Children's Hospital relentlessly to get the special formula for Sheila. She must have put so much faith in the diet but was now realising that Sheila was not going to get better and had to accept that she could no longer continue to look after her **and** her sons. It was just too stressful. Sheila was now nine years old, bigger and stronger but her mental age was no more than two years with increasingly difficult behaviour. She was very strong willed. The family were living in very poor accommodation in their back-to-back house at Aston and it was clear from social care records that things were exceedingly difficult for Mary as a single parent with four sons and a severely handicapped daughter to look after. It cannot have been easy to give up the struggle, and Sheila's admission to an NHS mental hospital would have been the only available option for Mary; she had no funds for any alternative care. There would be little or no understanding from the social care services at that time about how best to meet Sheila's needs for

10. Sheila at Chelmsley Hospital

the future, especially in the midst of such difficult family circumstances, and they would not have been aware that she had PKU or, indeed, known what that meant. Some idea of just how difficult it would have been to look after Sheila, prior to her admission, and how it must have impacted on the whole family is revealed in her records (extracted from her clinical notes at the time of her admission):

> *At the present time she* (i.e. Mary) *is unable to give the patient the necessary care and supervision she requires and has requested that she should be admitted informally to a mental deficiency hospital.*
>
> *Apparently normal at birth, no epilepsy and unable to speak. She was completely incontinent, unable to dress herself; she could drink from a cup but not able to feed herself with a spoon. Dribbles most of the time and mutters. Bawls and shouts for no apparent reason. Uncooperative. Walked at four years.*
>
> *Doesn't understand simple commands.*
>
> *She is a very retarded child with mental function at the age of a two year old. Easily upset and needs constant general psychiatric supervision as her lack of understanding could be a grave danger.*

The last statement referred to danger to Sheila herself; she had a total lack of awareness to potential danger and her brothers recall that she didn't seem to feel pain. After two weeks it was commented by the staff at Chelmsley that Sheila walked around aimlessly for long periods doing nothing and was unable to occupy herself and needed full care and attention. This was a very grim picture of how life was for Sheila at the time of her admission. She had never been to school and was recorded as 'uneducable'. This graphic description of her limited abilities emphasises the difficulties which Mary had been facing looking after her daughter in the family home. It was a credit to Mary that Sheila was well nourished and in good general health and she had been able to keep Sheila at home for so long with virtually no help. She was a caring mother.

On her admission to Chelmsley it was noted that Sheila had spent several periods as an inpatient at Birmingham Children's Hospital and had subsequently attended as an outpatient under Professor Squires at Little Bromwich Hospital. There was a passing mention of Phenylketonuria in the records in November 1959 – maybe Mrs Jones mentioned it. It was probably assumed to be of no relevance to Sheila's care at that time, after all there was no established treatment for PKU and likely there would be no other patients known to have PKU in the hospital, albeit there may have been some individuals whose diagnosis was not known. There was no mention of the dietary treatment trial undertaken at BCH in the early 1950s and no specific reference to the potential significance of Sheila's diagnosis and the fact was not mentioned again. Her PKU was just not seen as relevant to her care at that time. This would be the situation for many others with PKU (mostly undiagnosed cases) in similar institutions across the UK in the 1950s and 60s.

At the time of Sheila's admission the three eldest brothers were in a children's home, and when they came home Sheila was not there and never came to live at home again. Mary said very little to explain where Sheila had gone, she just said she was in hospital. It was her way of protecting her sons. There was a social stigma in those days about mental retardation so we imagine very little would have been said to others about where Sheila had gone. However Mary was very friendly with her next door neighbour, Peggy, and confided in her about Sheila. Trevor recalls his Mum using the word *'retarded'* to describe Sheila to Peggy but to everyone else the situation was simply not talked about.

The Early Years at Chelmsley

Terry: *'I think we knew how bad she was and she couldn't be at home'.*

Sheila was cared for in a large dormitory style ward with about 30-35 other children. Although the original block where she had lived was demolished as part of the redevelopment of the site in the 1990s, the new development includes some

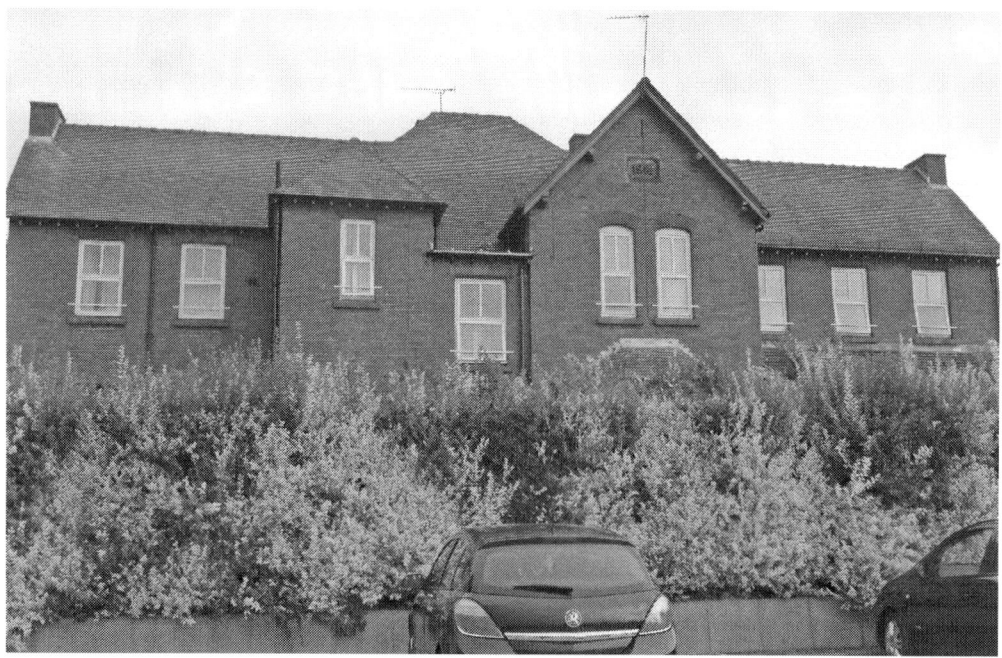

Former Chelmsley Hospital 2019 – Ward Block.

remains of the original hospital, with this block shown opposite being similar to the ward where Sheila lived.

As well as the wards the block contained kitchens, personal care areas and rows of bathrooms and toilets. Sheila's life was institutionalised as it was for the other patients and her day would be a fairly rigid routine, dominated by meals. Between meals, patients would transfer from the wards for periods to the day centre/leisure centre where there were various regular activities.

In spite of the continued pressures on Mary at home with four sons to care for she used to visit Sheila regularly at Chelmsley every month for about one to two hours each time. In those early days visits were not an automatic right – Mary had to apply in advance for a pass to visit and a car park pass (for the voluntary worker who would take her) for a specific date. This was done on her behalf by a case worker at the Birmingham Family Services Unit (FSU). The FSUs were formed in 1948 with the primary aim of helping families in difficulty in the aftermath of WWII. Their role was to promote the welfare of families and communities and the agency is identified as having a specific method of working focused on 'casework' with individuals and families. By the early 1960s Mary was receiving some support from a case worker 'Dorothy' with the Birmingham FSU who used to visit the home regularly and arrange the hospital visits for Mary. The brothers describe how Mary used to take Sheila a flask of tea and biscuits whenever she visited. When Mary arrived Sheila would gulp the tea down and then in Mary's own words *'scarper off'* so that she might only see Sheila for a few minutes. Sheila liked to be on her own. She loved her food and ate well.

The brothers did not visit regularly and describe how they were scared and upset by the surroundings at Chelmsley; Sheila could not speak and did not know who they were, she would run off when they arrived. They did not understand what was happening to their sister and it was very confusing, upsetting and frightening for the brothers. One of Sheila's younger brothers, Liam, recalls his Mum taking him with her to visit when he was only a young boy – he wasn't supposed to visit as such a young child – *'the surroundings used to scare me'*.

Visit Home 1963

By 1961, less than two years after Sheila's admission, Mary was beginning to think about whether Sheila could come home. Clearly Mary was feeling better in herself and very much wanted to look after Sheila at home. She made an application in March 1961 for her to be discharged from Chelmsley. The family were still living at the back-to-back house in Aston and the arrangement proposed was that Mary, Sheila now 11 years of age, and the two younger brothers would occupy the one bedroom and the other two older boys would have the attic. The

Sheila

application was turned down on the grounds it was felt Mary would not be able to give the care and supervision that would be needed for Sheila at that time. It must have been a huge disappointment to Mary. It was around this time that Mary made contact with one of her sisters in Ireland to ask her to visit; the brothers have vague memories of their Auntie coming to stay for a short period on this one occasion to visit the family in Aston, but this was the extent of the family contact.

Undaunted and a persistent Mary applied again in July 1963 – this time for Sheila to have just a visit home rather than discharged. The social worker felt it would be good for both Mary and Sheila and this time it was agreed that Sheila be granted leave for a home visit. The two elder boys would be away on a camping holiday in the summer holidays so the house at Victoria Road would be less crowded. Maybe Mary had plans and wishes that in the longer term perhaps Sheila could come home to live, meanwhile this short visit was allowed. Sheila was home for about six weeks.

The photograph below shows Sheila, now 13 years old, with her two younger brothers, Philip and Liam, during this visit home. They used to play at the rear of

Sheila with her brothers Philip (left) and Liam (right), 1963 (photograph kindly provided by the Jones Family).

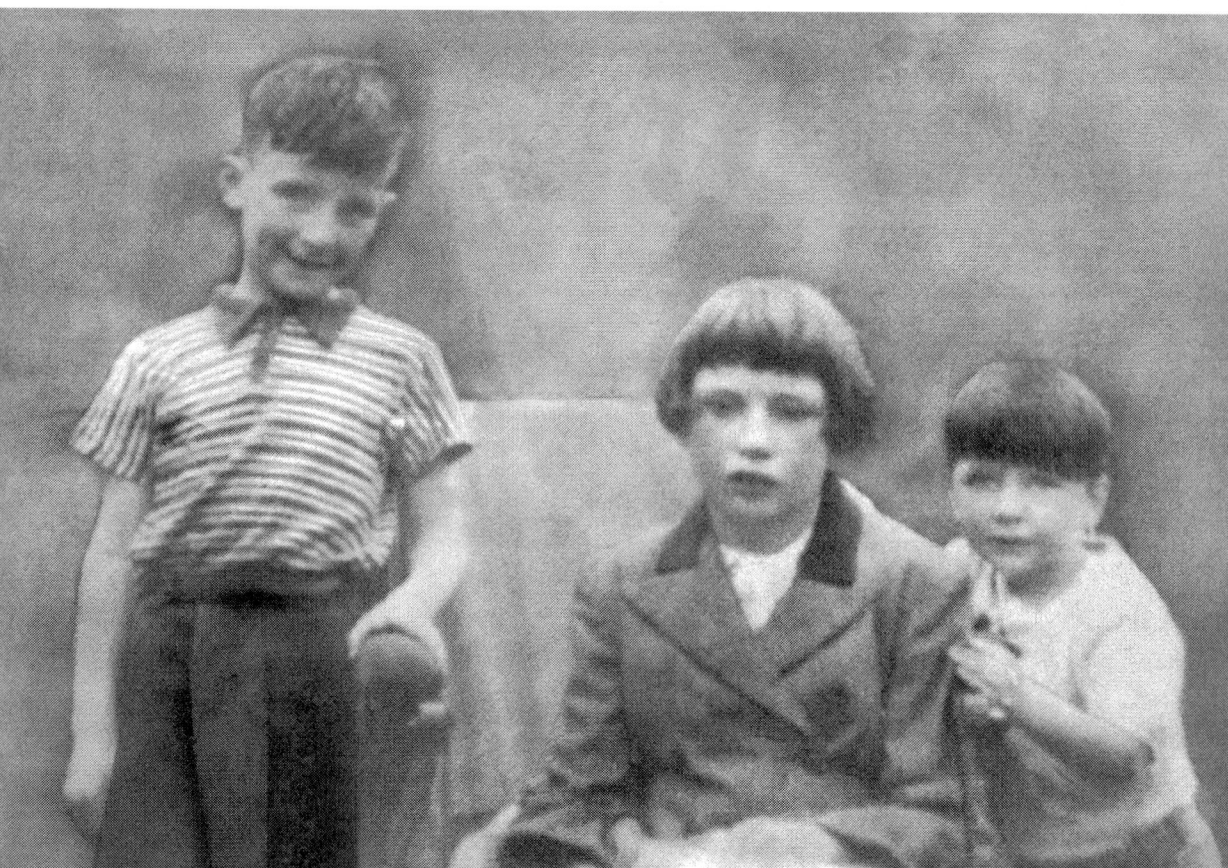

10. Sheila at Chelmsley Hospital

the back-to-backs in Victoria Road in a 'bombed out' derelict area. The youngest brother, Liam had previously never had the opportunity to get to know Sheila and Philip had only been five years of age when Sheila went to live at Chelmsley. They talk fondly about their memories of Sheila on this visit: *'She was dressed in her best coat with a velvet collar'*. Liam continues: *'I got to know Sheila quite well although I was only about four years old'*. They loved their sister.

Things however were difficult during this brief visit – Sheila's behaviour caused considerable disruption and problems at the family home. Sheila broke a window by throwing a brick at the next door neighbour. She was very strong willed and physically strong, and would run off at speed. This must have been heartbreaking for Mary as she realised that she couldn't look after Sheila at home. Sheila never returned home again.

Sheila and Mary

We don't know much about what life was like for Sheila when she returned to Chelmsley after this visit home in 1963 but records suggest that she seemed happier than previously – clapping and laughing at times. Her general health continued to be good and she had begun to settle down into a routine. She continued to be completely incapable of looking after herself, and guarding her from common dangers was a continued concern. One early behavioural issue was that Sheila kept taking her clothes off. However, with time and patience from the staff she did learn that she needed to stay dressed: again with the help of staff she also ceased to be incontinent. She still had no speech and communication continued to be a major issue. Her behaviour became more of a problem during the 1970s and she became challenging and aggressive at times. Sheila didn't like contact with others and preferred her own company and disliked any disturbance to her routine. Overall, however, there had been some small improvement, albeit slow, in Sheila's skills. She was fully mobile, although she always walked on her tip toes and wore special boots, and was, in fact, able to move very quickly when she wanted to. She was now able to dress and undress herself with persuasion, patience

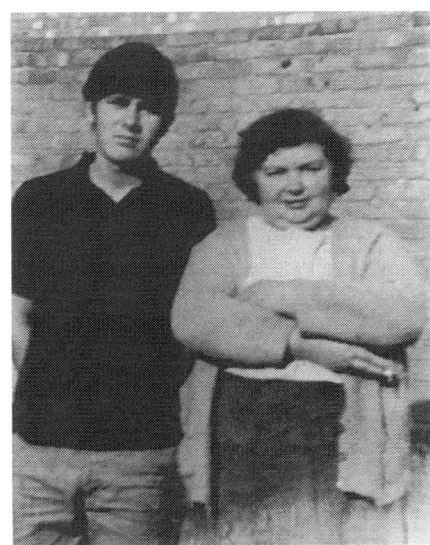

Sheila's brother Trevor and Mary at Aston, 1960s (photograph kindly provided by the Jones Family).

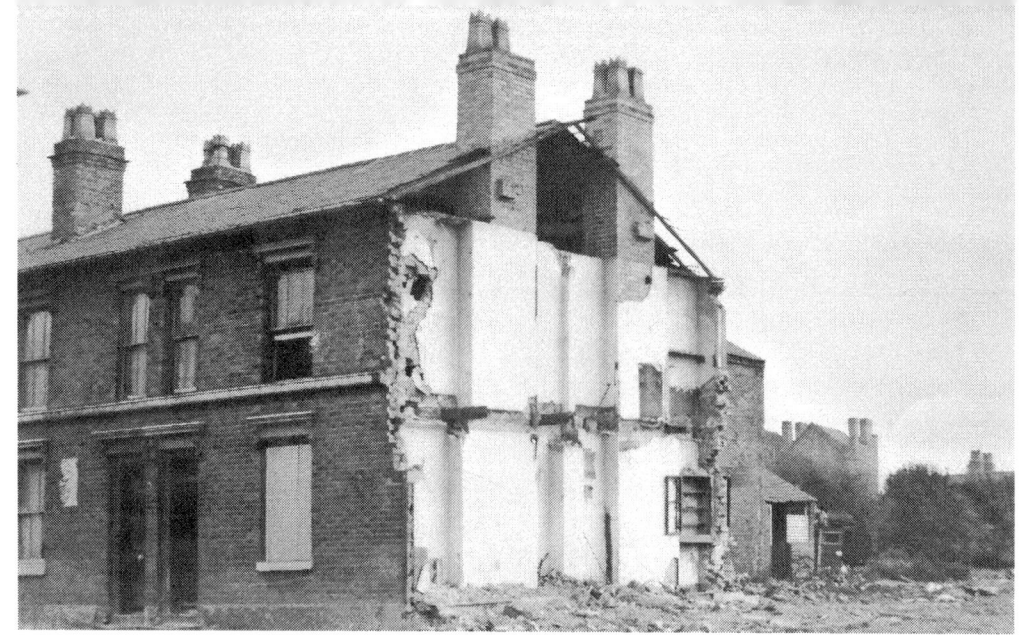

Demolition of houses at Victoria Road, Aston, c.1968 (photograph courtesy of Birmingham Libraries).

and time from the staff. She continued to eat well and feed herself with a spoon and drank from a cup; she still loved her tea! She began to have some independence and would clearly express her dislike of something if it didn't suit.

During this time Mary had continued to live at Victoria Road with her four sons.

After further treatment for her stress she had recovered well. She kept the family together until the late 1960s when the back-to-back houses at Victoria road were finally demolished to make way for the new expressway into the city. They were one of the last families to move out as the houses around them were vacated and demolished.

Trevor moved away, and Mary with Terry, Philip and Liam moved to Perry Common in north Birmingham. In 1971 Mary was well and attended Trevor's wedding.

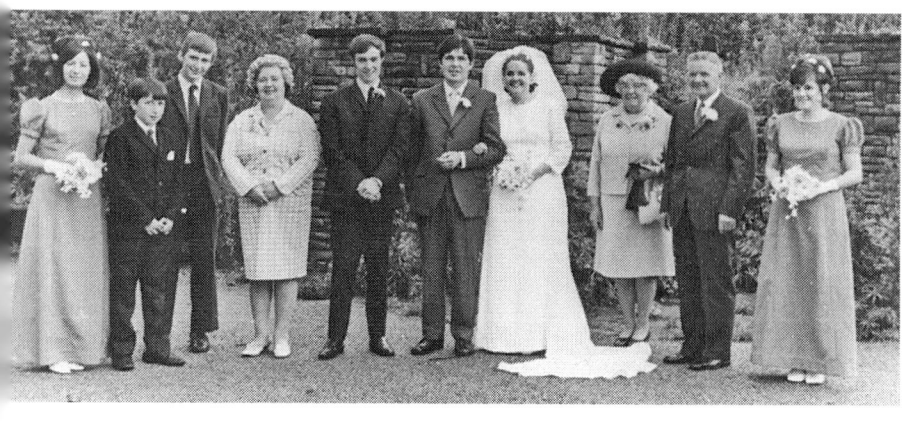

Mary Jones at Trevor (Sheila's brother) and Marilyn's wedding 1971 in Birmingham (photograph kindly provided by the Jones Family.

Mary continued to visit Sheila on a regular basis, now making the journey from north Birmingham over to Chelmsley on the bus and was still visiting in 1980. Sheila was now 30 years of age and there were now few children at Chelmsley as most, like Sheila, had become long term patients and had reached adulthood; children were no longer being admitted. Mary became unwell during the late 1970s with fewer visits to see Sheila and sadly died aged 64 years in 1981 from cancer and was buried at Witton cemetery in north Birmingham. Mary had continued her regular visits to see Sheila at Chelmsley for over 20 years. Sheila was in Mary's heart until the day she died.

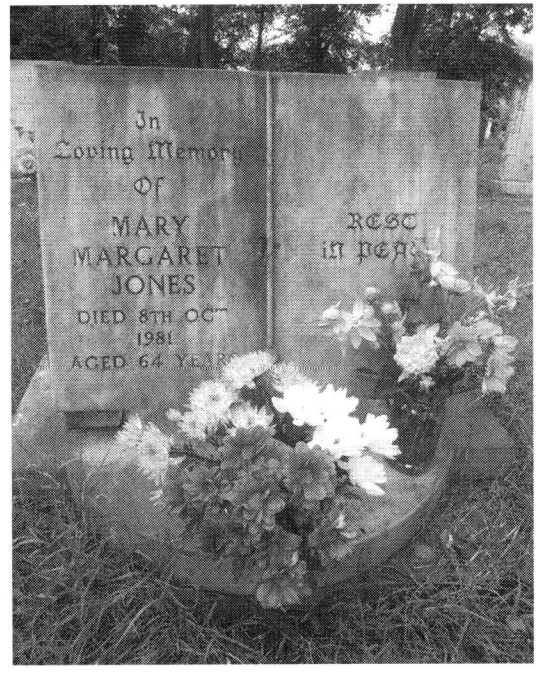

Mary's Grave, north Birmingham.

Sheila after her Mum

After her Mum died, Sheila had little contact with her family. She did not know who her brothers were and didn't want to spend time with them. Terry visited a couple of times but sadly she did not recognise him. There were few visitors for any of the patients at Chelmsley but that was not unusual as there was a stigma and a fear associated with mental hospitals. Sheila's life was now totally in the hands of the dedicated staff at Chelmsley. For many years she was looked after by Dr Brian Oliver, Consultant Psychiatrist. Several of the staff who cared for Sheila at Chelmsley from the late 1970s and through the 1980s and early 1990s are long serving dedicated staff and are still working at the Hospital (Brooklands, see p.81). They have helped create a picture of Sheila's life in Gorse Ward.

The ward had about 35 female patients with a wide range of disabilities, many severe, and it was a demanding place to work with few nurses. In the early years perhaps, at best, there were only three staff members for each 12 hour shift. The same staff would do everything from bathing and dressing patients, polishing shoes, washing clothes, serving meals, making beds and supervising various activities. Each morning from 6.30am to 9.30am they would bath, dress and give the patients breakfast. It was non-stop back breaking work. Food was prepared on site in a centralised kitchen and then distributed to the wards on large trolleys. Tea was dispensed using enormous teapots. Main items for washing such as bedding were sent to the centralised laundry on site, but the ward had a twin tub washing machine where nurses would wash the smaller items such as socks, underwear etc. Occasionally the ward would have a helper from the Youth Training Scheme (YTS). This was a government scheme in the 1980s for young school leavers to gain some work experience, perhaps prior to formal training to be a nurse. The YTS workers would help to make the 35 beds every day and help dressing the patients. It was sheer hard work.

Sheila would require help with everything. Her main problem was communication. She could not speak and never uttered any words but vocalised a lot with a variety of sounds making her wishes known. A high pitched squeal was associated with elation and excitement whereas more of a growl told everyone she was not happy. The same staff were regularly on the ward so got to know her moods well from these sounds; new staff wouldn't understand at first but soon learnt. Sheila generally seemed happy but could be grumpy at times. Staff remarked that she was a very determined lady and knew what she wanted and what she didn't want, a characteristic which many have commented on. The earliest memories from the staff was of Sheila in the 1970s (now in her 20s) – *'a pretty young lady with shoulder length fair hair – well-nourished'*, described as *'meaty'*, and looked well.

Sheila wasn't for staying in bed and liked her bath and would brush her own hair. After the morning routine Sheila and others would be taken out from the ward block, usually in a small group, with two staff to the WRVS

Staff at Brooklands Hospital

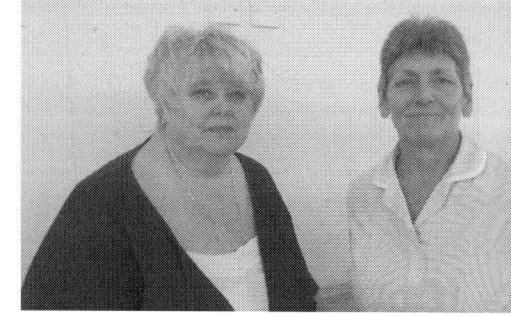

Lynn (left) and Angela (right), 2016.

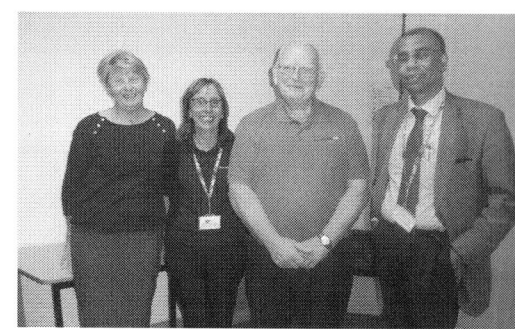

From left to right: The Author with Staff (Maggie, Derek and Dr Ashok Roy), 2019.

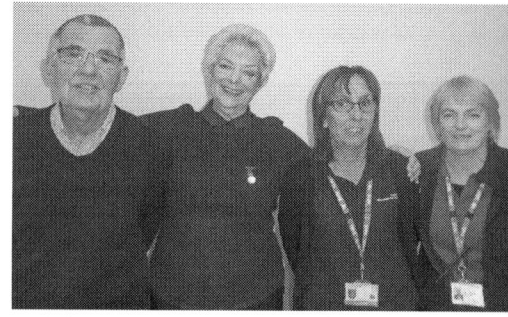

From left to right: Trevor Jones with Staff (Theresa, Maggie and Carol), 2019.

(Womens Royal Voluntary Service) canteen to get more food (usually cakes!), where on a Friday everyone would get a cream cake. This was a real treat. Then they would go to the leisure centre or recreation building (known as the 'Rec') for various activities for an hour or so. Some patients, depending on their ability, were able to go to the hospital workshop (Light Industrial Unit or LIU) during the day to undertake simple tasks such as placing small components in bags; they enjoyed this and it gave them a purpose. All patients would attend the regular activities, including those in wheelchairs and those who, like Sheila could not fully participate – everyone was included. Then it was back to the ward for lunch. If weather permitted the afternoon would be a walk around the grounds or the garden; Gorse Ward had a garden at the back. Sheila loved going outside and sometimes got the occasional sunburn. She loved the sun on her face and would turn towards it when it was shining through the window. At other times she would just wander around the ward area and wait for her meals. Then it was eating again with the evening meal before night school. This consisted of various activities including floristry, crochet, music, drawing and cooking. Again Sheila would go to these activities, even though she could not necessarily participate. The hospital's philosophy was about the opportunity to be together with others. By 9pm it was bath time and then bed. The staff would go home exhausted after 12 hours on duty and sometimes longer.

As well as the usual daytime routine there were lots of additional on-site events on a regular basis. Sheila would be taken to the 'pictures' (cinema) on a Wednesday and 'disco' on a Friday night in the 'Rec'. Sunday there was a Church service where some of the patients would be allowed to play musical instruments. Sometimes there was bingo session, and a pantomime at Christmas. Bonfire night was another special event for everyone. Sheila would also go to the hairdresser; there was a salon in one of the other wards. She would have sessions in the on-site swimming baths. She loved her food, especially ice cream, and would have the special treat of cream cakes on Fridays as well as fish and chips. On more than one occasion she was caught climbing through the hatch into the ward kitchen.

A set of clean clothes for each patient was put out as a 'bundle' every morning. Each patient had a clothing order for new clothes twice a year, for a summer and a winter wardrobe. There was a monetary allowance and a specific member of staff was designated to undertake this and shop for six patients, usually to Marks and Spencer in Birmingham city centre. Sheila showed no interest in her clothes but nevertheless was provided with a new set each year.

Day trips were a feature of life at Chelmsley in the 1970s and 1980s. These were wide ranging including regular trips to adventure parks, Charlecote Park to see the deer and the riverside at Stratford-upon-Avon. These trips were important and would be something of interest to break up the routine of an institutionalised life. The hospital had its own mobility bus with a driver who would take about eight patients together with two members of staff. They sometimes even went as far as the seaside from land locked Birmingham to Weston-super-Mare. The bus would leave as soon as breakfast was over with a two to three hour drive to the coast where they would all have a picnic and then drive back again. It would be 8pm before they were home to the hospital and then bath and bedtime. Sheila loved the mini bus trips and got very excited when they took place. There was one notable occasion when towards the end of a day trip to Drayton Manor Park (an adventure park), Sheila was being pushed in a wheelchair (she was tired) when she suddenly jumped out of the wheelchair to her feet and ran towards a family who had just bought 'Mr Whippy' ice creams with huge long pointed swirls on top of the wafer cone. The nurse recalls how *'Sheila pinched the ice cream from the top of the cone and shoved it in her mouth!',* and how she had to buy a replacement ice cream for the rather bewildered family. Sheila had a contented happy look on her face which spoke volumes: *'that's all I needed I am quite happy to go home now'.*

With such large numbers of patients at Chelmsley and limited staff, help from volunteers was an important contribution to the care of the patients. Chelmsley had 1:1 days when a volunteer would come for the day to befriend a particular patient. There were also schemes for students to help, in particular during the summer holidays, with foreign exchange students who used to come and stay on site and help take the patients out. It was valuable work experience for the students and in turn enriched the lives of the patients.

Another special event which took place every year was the Jumbo run when a group of volunteer motorcyclists came with motor bikes with side cars and would take the patients out; Sheila would sit in the side car for her day out. The voluntary organisation (Jumbo GB), working with those with disabilities and special needs, has a long standing association with Chelmsley as evidenced by the annual trips which took place:

1973 Chelmsley Hospital to Ragley Hall
1974 Chelmsley Hospital to Twycross Zoo
1975 Chelmsley Hospital to Twycross Zoo
1976 Chelmsley Hospital to West Midlands Safari Park
1977 Chelmsley Hospital to Billing Aquadrome
1978 Chelmsley Hospital to Twycross Zoo
1979 Chelmsley Hospital to Cosford
1980 Chelmsley Hospital Green to Billing Aquadrome

10. Sheila at Chelmsley Hospital

1981 Chelmsley Hospital Green to Candeys Circus
1982 Chelmsley Hospital Green to Hewell Grange
1983 Chelmsley Hospital to Black Country Museum
1984 Chelmsley Hospital to Bass Charington Museum

Chelmsley Staff member: *'It was quite a sight to see a convoy of bikes setting off with road closures and a police escort – this would end in everyone enjoying a massive picnic and having a really good fun day out'.*

Sometimes the whole ward would be taken on holiday, as far as Colwyn Bay in North Wales, Teignmouth in Devon or even Jersey, one of the Channel Islands. It would be unthinkable today. These activities provided much needed enrichment and colour to the otherwise institutionalised patients' daily routine which today could not be envisaged. It is of considerable comfort to know that Sheila was included in these activities, the staff recalling that her last holiday was in rural Wales. These trips must have provided much happiness and fun for her over her many years being cared for at Chelmsley.

By the late 1980s Sheila's care had been taken over by Dr Ashok Roy, Consultant Psychiatrist. The hospital had continued to change and by now Gorse Ward was entirely adult female and most individuals had severe disabilities, as many with less severe problems had been discharged from the hospital. Gorse became one of the wards housing patients with the most challenging behaviours to manage and Dr Roy describes the pressures for the medical staff at that time with such a high intensity of demanding patients. There were still over 700 patients at Chelmsley and only three medical consultants, as was the situation in those days for the Mental Health Services. He remembers Sheila as not easy and quite volatile and vocal; she was a determined lady and knew her own mind. By now fewer opportunities for activities and day trips were available to patients as new rules and regulations came into practice. The hospital farm and workshop had closed down and there was less of interest for patients to occupy their time. This made it more difficult to manage those with severe challenging behaviour as boredom became problematic.

Sheila 1987

Although Sheila was living at Chelmsley from 1959 nothing further was known to the 'PKU world' about her whereabouts after 1955/6 until 1987. Her life at Chelmsley was not known about to those elsewhere and she had essentially got lost in the 'system' for over 30 years. Mental Health Services, especially the large institutions/former asylums were not integrated with the rest of the health service.

By the 1970s the practice of screening all newborn infants for PKU had been introduced nationwide (see p.91) and the benefits of the dietary treatment for the early treated cases, diagnosed following screening, was now well established. At that time it was considered as a treatment of limited duration during early childhood whilst the brain was still developing. Continuing beyond this age was practically very difficult to achieve in school aged children and some thought the unpleasant diet to be associated with emotional disturbances. It had therefore become practice to discontinue the diet in early childhood at around the age of five or six years of age. In the UK it was initially recommended that diet could be discontinued at eight years of age but by the late 1970s the advice had changed to remain on treatment throughout childhood (Smith et al 1978). Concerns were emerging about deterioration in cognitive function if the diet was stopped earlier. By the mid-1980s the practice of most clinics was discontinuation of diet in late childhood. It was, at that time, not considered as of being of benefit during adulthood in an already severely affected individual like Sheila.

Research had shown that phenylalanine was actively transported across the placenta and could damage the developing baby. As the first cohorts from the newborn screening programmes reached child bearing age, having discontinued diet at an early age, it became recognised that untreated PKU causes great risk of adverse effects to the unborn foetus. By the 1980s these risks had been confirmed and in order to protect the developing baby, a phenylalanine restricted diet was now recommended during pregnancy. This was an emerging issue for PKU individuals who had come off diet and were no longer actively being followed up. In addition there were individuals with undiagnosed and untreated PKU (i.e. females of child bearing age who pre-dated newborn screening) being cared for in mental institutions. For this reason in the 1980s the BCH Inherited Metabolic Disorders laboratory was encouraging investigation of mentally retarded females who were still of child bearing age because of the potential risk of pregnancy from untreated PKU. As part of this initiative, the laboratory received blood and urine samples for investigation for PKU from several female patients being cared for in the various mental institutions which still existed around Birmingham. In 1987 a blood sample from a 37 year old lady, Sheila Jones, at Chelmsley Hospital arrived. The sample had very high levels of phenylalanine and PKU was confirmed in the patient. This was a previously unknown case to the service. The early publication on PKU treatment by Dr Bickel et al from BCH in 1954 had the identity 'Sh.Jo.' on the illustrations and the laboratory wondered if this could be the same person. After contacting the medical staff at Chelmsley Hospital it was established this was indeed the same Sheila Jones who had been treated at BCH in 1951; the fact that she had PKU had been 'lost'/disregarded in her mental health records. The IMD team at BCH engaged with Sheila's carers at Chelmsley and were able to meet her in 1987.

10. Sheila at Chelmsley Hospital

Sheila still had no speech although she understood simple commands; she had major communication and behaviour problems and was functioning at the level of severe mental retardation. Seeing Sheila with her severe disabilities was sad and a stark reminder, particularly to those involved with the successes of newborn screening, of what untreated PKU meant.

It was increasingly becoming realised that a reduced phenylalanine diet might be of some benefit to late treated PKUs in helping with their behaviour and how they felt e.g. mood, anxiety levels. The metabolic team from BCH discussed with the medical team caring for Sheila the possible benefits of introducing a low phenylalanine diet to see if it might help Sheila in any way. It was decided to try and great efforts were made, but it proved not possible to implement any meaningful dietary change. Sheila was not able to cooperate and it was too distressing to continue with no real certainty of any benefit.

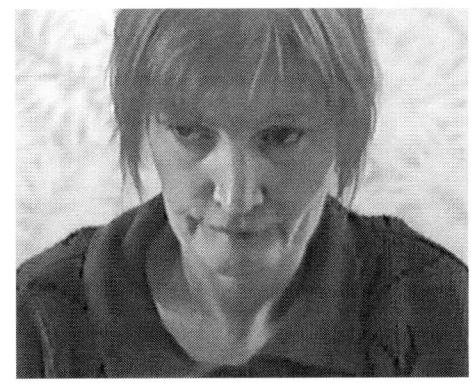

Sheila in 1987 aged 37 years at Chelmsley Hospital (photograph reproduced courtesy of the Jones Family).

In the mid-1980s Sheila had begun to have medical problems unrelated to her PKU. She started to refuse food, vomit and lose weight. Problems concerning her gastrointestinal (GI) tract developed and eating became a real difficulty for her. Unfortunately, these problems became chronic in spite of various attempts of treatments to alleviate them. In addition to these GI issues Sheila's mental health deteriorated and she became very disturbed with more challenging behaviour. Sheila continued to be looked after at Chelmsley and for several more years continued to feed and dress herself, but sadly her GI problems persisted and became more severe.

Brooklands

As part of the reorganisation of Mental Health Services to provide more community-based services across the UK, the majority of the Chelmsley residents were discharged or went to live in the community (see Appendix III). Brooklands Hospital was built in the early 1990s for patients from Chelmsley who continued to require hospital-based care. It is a purpose built NHS unit for adults and children with learning disabilities and is part of the NHS Mental Health Services. It currently houses approximately 60 residents. It was built as a

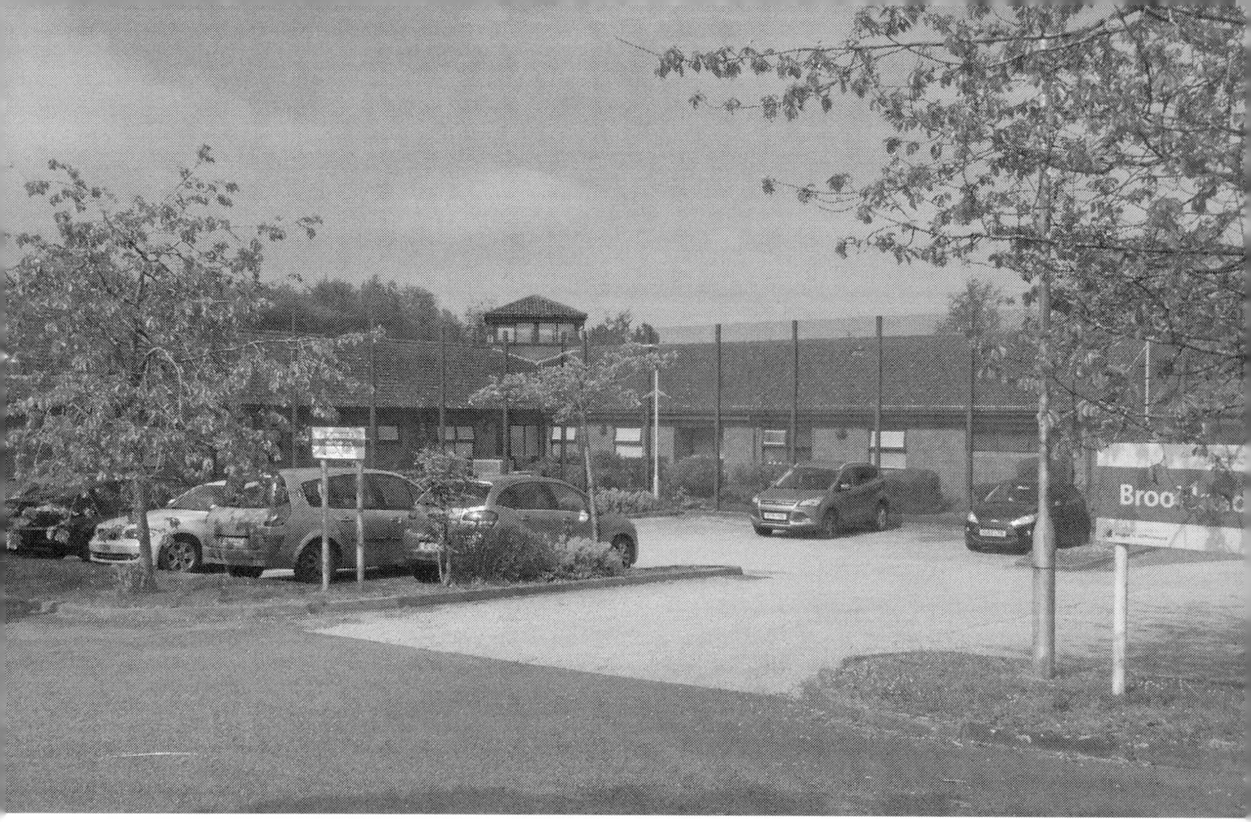

Brooklands Hospital 2019.

series of separate units, bungalow style, each accommodating up to five to six residents. The impetus behind this change was to make living as normal as possible with a high quality of both environment and clinical care. Brooklands is located adjacent to the original Chelmsley Hospital which was subsequently partly demolished and redeveloped.

Sheila was transferred to Brooklands around the mid-1990s. In contrast to Chelmsley this provided a non-institutionalised 'homely' environment where Sheila lived semi-domestic style with four or five other patients in Bungalow Seven. She would have a routine day of fairly 'normal' activities including trips out two or

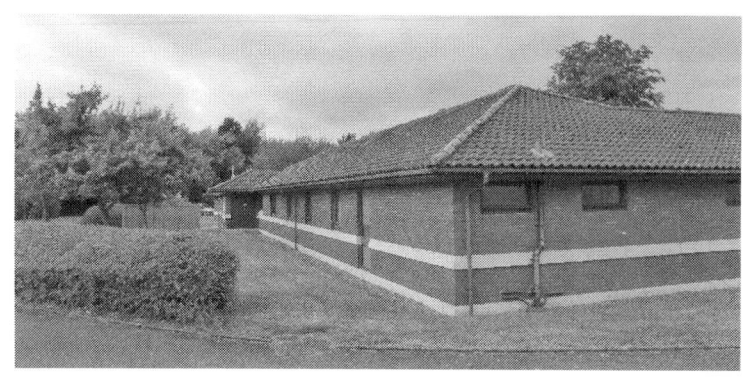

Bungalow Unit at Brooklands Hospital, 2019.

three times each week to shops, sometimes a bus ride, and to other places for relaxation and interest. Sheila really liked to go out and because she had been admitted on an 'informal' basis, she was not in any way restricted in her activities. Although the exact bungalow where Sheila lived is no longer in use, similar buildings are part of the current complex.

Reflections from the Staff at Chelmsley/Brooklands

Staff member at Brooklands Hospital, West Midlands (2016): *'We should be proud of Sheila – in her own way she helped so many'.*

Sheila was like many who lived at Chelmsley, a long standing patient well known to the staff. The staff speak about her with great affection and said she was a *'real character'*. Although she had no speech, *'she was strong and could defend herself if there was something she didn't want to do. She knew what she liked and what she didn't like, and was a very determined lady'*; this characteristic was repeated again and again by so many who knew her. She did have a temper at times and sometimes got quite angry. She didn't like contact with people and didn't like to be touched. She had no particular friends and although she liked her own solitude she would often spend time 'on her own' but in the same vicinity with others who liked to do the same. In the ward she spent most of the time on her own; *'she used to rock a lot and looked sad at times'*. However, *'she would initiate contact if she wanted you for something. She could feed herself but liked you to help her dress her'*. She loved her food but later had to have everything minced because of her GI problems. The staff particularly remember her love of tea.

> *'You could not put a cup of tea down because Sheila would pinch it!'*
> *'She used to run on her tip toes and had special boots and would "scoot" up the ward at great speed'.*
> *'She was a lovable character – I loved her to pieces'.*
> *'I can still see her scooting through the ward'.*
> *'Used to have a song sang to her – she liked that – she would smile'.*
> *'She would drink her tea and didn't want to know you after that!'*
> *'Used to pinch other people's tea – can see her if you turned your back'.*

Sheila – A Tribute

Sadly, Sheila deteriorated with worsening liver function. In spite of intensive investigation and management for her gastro intestinal problems, she died aged 49 years at Brooklands on 29th January 1999. Her funeral took place on 19th February at the church of Our Lady Help of Christians, Birmingham where the following tribute was read (BCH Archive):

A TRIBUTE TO SHEILA

– given by Anne Green on 19th February 1999 at the Church of Our Lady Help of Christians, Birmingham

First of all I would like to introduce myself. I am Anne Green and I am here with one of my colleagues Kate Hall from the Children's Hospital in Birmingham. We wanted to be here to join you all today with Sheila's family, friends and carers to pay tribute and celebrate Sheila's life.

I first came to know Sheila in 1986 and met her in 1987 because of my work and interest in a disorder called phenylketonuria. It was in 1987 that I came to know that she was a very special person. Sheila had this condition and it was responsible for her handicap from a very early age. I would like to take few minutes to explain the significance of Sheila's history.

At the age of 17 months Sheila was already retarded and in 1951 she was taken to the Children's Hospital where she was found to have phenylketonuria, the first child to be diagnosed with this condition in Birmingham. There was no treatment for this disorder – however doctors at the Children's Hospital had an idea that a special type of diet might be able to correct the problem. They set about producing a diet and later that year in September 1951 she was admitted to the Children's Hospital to try this diet. This showed that the diet could reduce the chemicals in Sheila's blood which were causing her handicap and might have a beneficial effect. On the basis of Sheila's trial the treatment for PKU was developed across the world and in the 1960's it was possible to obtain these diets commercially. By 1970 its success was proven and now all newborn babies virtually across the whole world are tested for PKU and if affected treatment starts from birth. Sadly, Sheila and other patients at that time were unable to benefit but now every year about 70 new babies in the UK diagnosed with PKU are treated and grow up normally. Sadly, Sheila never knew what had been achieved. It is very important that we all, doctors and other professionals working with PKU, children and families with PKU recognise and remember Sheila's contribution, her great 'gift' with her family and doctors at that time that so many others across the world now benefit. The history of Sheila's early years will live on, it is a land-mark and is recorded in the medical literature. I feel privileged to be here today and I know that I speak for other Biochemists, doctors, children and families with PKU to say our own thankyou to Sheila for her great gift to so many others.

Sheila is buried at Woodlands Cemetery on the east side of Birmingham, near to Chelmsley/Brooklands Hospital.

Her grave has a special epitaph which refers to the diet which she had. The importance of the treatment was sadly not for Sheila herself but the huge legacy she left for the benefit of everyone with PKU today. A dedication plaque in her memory is located at BCH in the Clinical Chemistry laboratory.

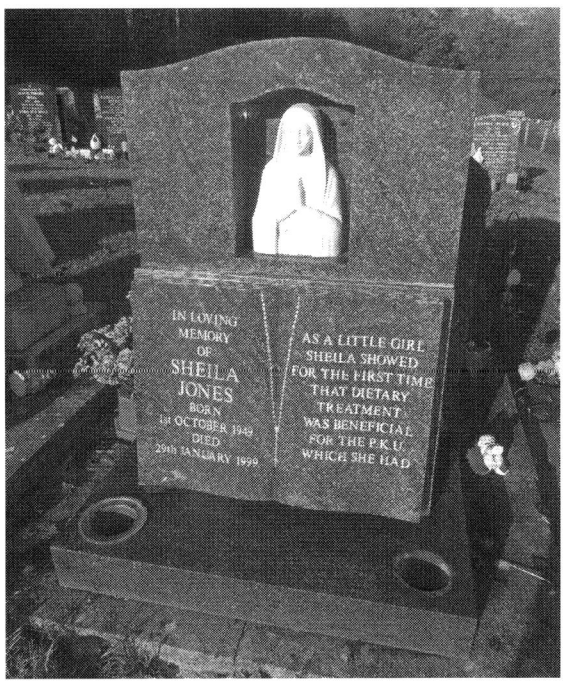

Sheila's Grave at Woodlands Cemetery, Birmingham 2019.

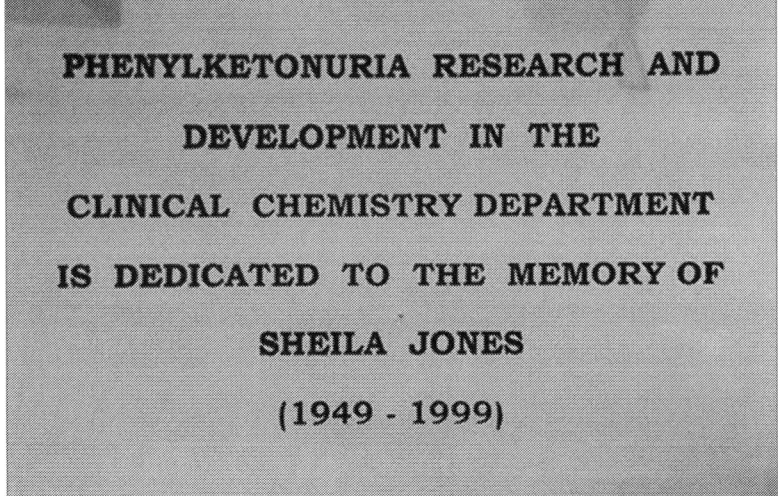

Dedication Plaque at BCH.

11

PKU DEVELOPMENTS

Since the pioneering treatment for Sheila the developments in the field of PKU have been huge. During the 40 years that Sheila was being cared for at Chelmsley/ Brooklands Hospital, services for PKU developed at a rapid pace both within the UK and beyond, much of which has been a direct result of her first dietary treatment.

Development of Commercial Protein Substitutes

Dr Hickmans: *'They* (newly diagnosed PKUs, c.1960) *are supplied with a low phenylalanine preparation in solid form. The trouble is that this "flour" is difficult to cook and very nasty to taste'.*

Production of the phenylalanine 'free' casein hydrolysate in the Birmingham laboratory clearly could not continue long term and there became an obvious and compelling need to provide diets for other patients. The scene had been set and provided stimulus for manufacture of the special mixture on a commercial basis. In 1954 Allen and Hanburys had provided the Birmingham team with a phenylalanine 'free' casein hydrolysate product for Sheila, so it would be around this date that the 'homemade' production in Dr Hickmans' lab would have been replaced by this commercially available source. Sheila's brothers refer to a *'powdery stuff in tins'* which would have been this first commercial product. This differed from the Birmingham laboratory 'mix' in that it was provided as a powder to dissolve in water.

Other hospitals in the UK were also beginning to treat patients. In a letter to the Chief Dietitian (Pam Griffiths) at Bristol Children's Hospital (23rd August 1954) Allen and Hanburys refer to the production of a 'casein hydrolysate of low phenylalanine content (<10mg/100g product)' – it was only available in restricted quantities and was expensive – at a cost of 170/- (shillings) per kg (£8.50/kg) – but not yet listed in the general catalogue. The understanding that the product could have a permissible 'low' phenylalanine content rather than be completely phenylalanine 'free' had greatly reduced the time required to produce and hence reduced the cost. The production, however, was described as 'somewhat limited' (Williams 1954).

11 PKU Developments

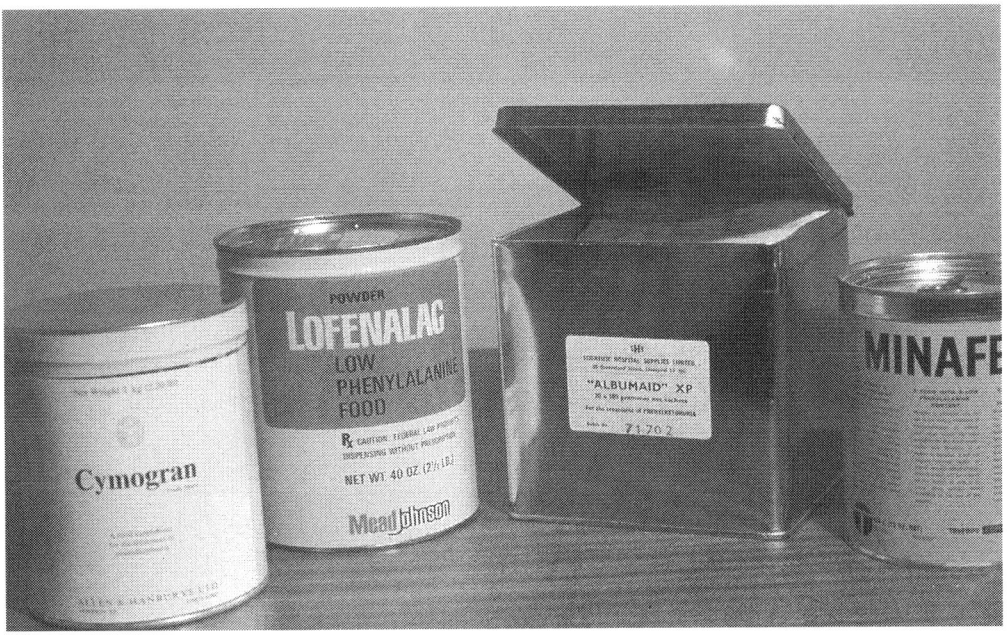

Cymogran, together with other early protein substitutes for PKU (photograph kindly provided by Christine Clothier).

Although a few PKU patients around the UK were beginning to receive this early product, it was still not available on prescription and there was some difficulty obtaining the material for outpatient use and concern about who would pay for it. The NHS was still only six years old. There was an increasing demand for their product and so Allen and Hanburys began to market 'Cymogran' which had evolved from the original formula prepared in Birmingham.

Another British firm Trufood then developed 'Minafen' specifically for infants, based on the work by Louis Woolf from Great Ormond Street in 1955. Two products were developed in America: 'Lofenalac' by Mead Johnson in 1958 and 'Ketonil' by Merck, Sharp and Dohme. In 1960 another protein substitute became available 'Albumaid XP', this time using hydrolysed albumin as the source of amino acids with phenylalanine removed. This was produced by Scientific Hospital Supplies (SHS) Ltd (formed in 1960 as a subsidiary of Powell and Scholefield Ltd) a pioneering company, based in Liverpool, producing special dietary products. SHS became synonymous with products for metabolic disorders in the UK for many decades. The close involvement between clinicians and the nutritional industry was an altruistic partnership and was the precursor to many therapeutic initiatives for uncommon 'orphan' disorders, not just PKU.

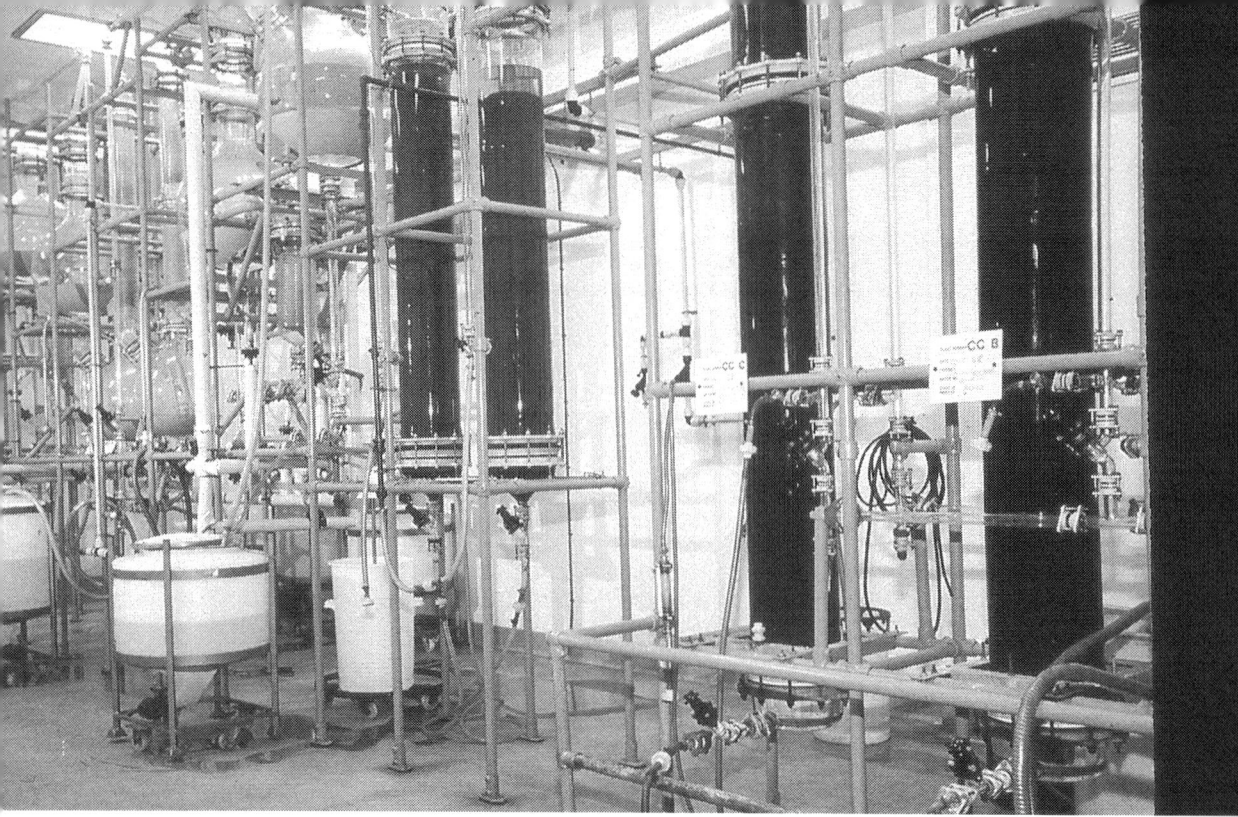

Commercial production of phenylalanine low <0.5mg/100g product) amino acid mixture using charcoal columns (Albumaid XP) (photograph kindly provided by Christine Clothier).

The commercial production by SHS used large industrial sized charcoal columns and was an order of magnitude greater than the 3 ft. long column used in the Birmingham laboratory.

Further Development of Diets and Paediatric Dietetics
Availability of more palatable phenylalanine 'free' protein substitutes, and help and support for PKU patients and their families to manage the diet, became a critical part of the next stages of development. These had not been available for Sheila and the other very early treated cases but would become essential if good long term control of diet was to be achieved.

The practical problem of producing an acceptable diet for babies and young infants was initially a major issue, and concerns over excessive restriction of phenylalanine and need for vitamin supplementation becoming evident with work from Birmingham and Exeter (Brimblecombe et al 1961). There was little if any information available for families and preparation of diets to restrict phenylalanine intake was limited by lack of knowledge of the phenylalanine content of many foods. There was little practical guidance on the construction of the diets and they remained monotonous and unpalatable owing to the unpleasant taste of the hydrolysate amino acid mixtures. As more information became available on the protein content of various foodstuffs, this allowed for more flexibility and was especially important for older children; the concept of 'exchanges' was established so patients and families could more easily manage their own diet. The development of metabolic dietetic services for children became crucial to the subsequent success of the treatment (Clothier 2019).

By 1964 commercial preparations were available on prescription and there were further advances in the 1970s and beyond to make the foods tastier and more palatable to take, with new recipes. Dietitians became an integral and essential part of the clinical metabolic team. Although there were now several phenylalanine free products available, they were not complete foods and had to be supplemented with the necessary carbohydrates, fats, vitamins and minerals. Creation of low protein recipes became an important skill and paved the way for manufacture of low protein products which could be used to improve the diet. Diets today and the taste of protein substitutes bear no resemblance to what Sheila and many others with PKU had to tolerate in the 1950s and 1960s.

Demonstrating the Effects of Dietary Treatment
It had become important to demonstrate the benefits of treatment on the development of the individual. Monitoring of patients with IQ measurements became part of their management. In 1958 Louis Woolf and colleagues reported their experience with their original three patients (followed for a further 32 months) and a further seven patients. In almost every case there was a sharp and significant rise in IQ associated with commencement of the diet although in one young infant, treated from five weeks of age IQ did not improve suggesting that damage had already occurred (Woolf et al 1958). This was overall very encouraging but emphasised the importance of very early diagnosis for the diet to be successful.

By 1960 the importance of early diagnosis and commencement of treatment was clearly shown. Data on 55 cases from England and the USA were compiled and published from Birmingham (Blainey and Squire 1960). This publication records the final mental development, expressed as IQ (or DQ), of all children reported in the literature to June 1960, including unpublished data from cases in England and America (see p.90). This work showed that the number of children who attain an IQ of over 60% declines steeply if the age of starting treatment is over one year whereas almost all those treated in the first few weeks of life, albeit a small number, have an IQ within the normal range.

In 1960 Dr Bickel, now in Marburg, reviewed his experiences over a nine year period, reporting on treatment of a further 10 patients and reviewed 79 cases reported by others (Bickel and Grueter 1960). There was no doubt that by giving

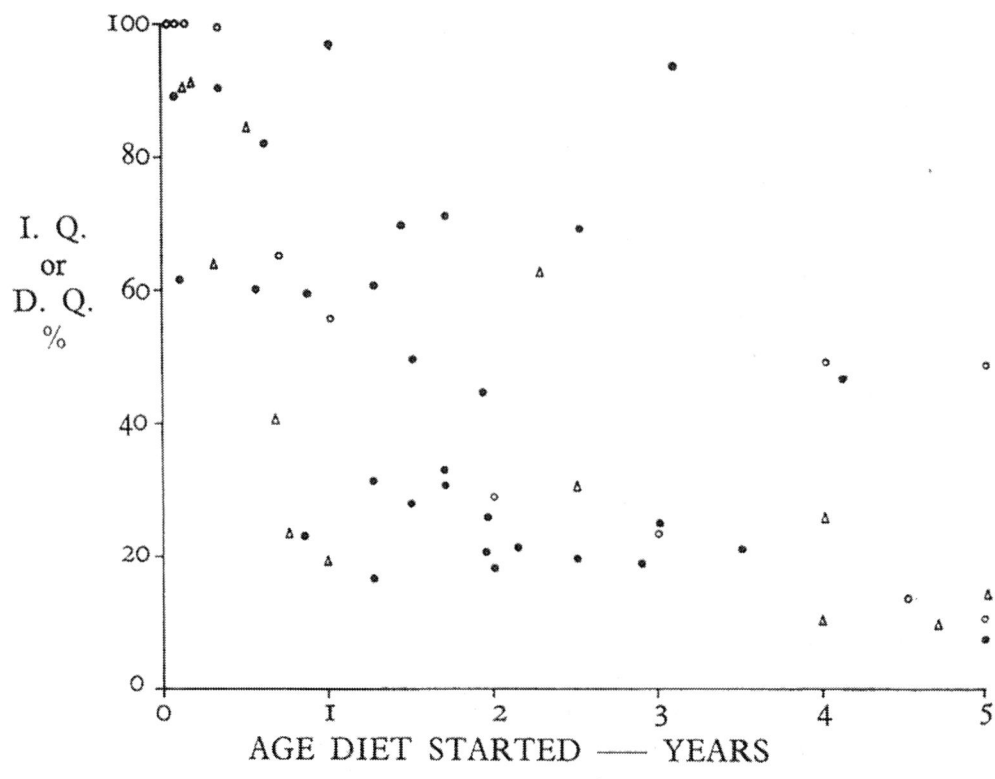

Relationship between final mental development recorded and the age of commencing dietary treatment in 55 PKU children (reproduced from Blainey. J.D. and Squire, J.R., 1961).

a low phenylalanine diet, normal blood levels could be achieved although daily intake of phenylalanine varied from case to case.

It was now becoming accepted that early diagnosis followed by dietary treatment can allow normal mental development in a least some cases with PKU. There were however many unanswered questions: it was unknown how long the diet would be required for and how tight the biochemical control needed to be. Measurement of mental development in each individual over a period of time would become critical in assessment of progress. There was also concern that not all cases might require treatment and that some might not respond to treatment. We now know much more about the existence of variant forms of PKU, transient cases of hyperphenylalaninaemia, mild hyperphenylalaninaemia and cofactor deficiency cases, which either do not require or do not respond to diet (p.109). All this was not known at that time so a lot of questions remained and there was quite rightly concern about the optimal policy. Even as late as 1967 there were advocates of the need for validation, of treatment with a diet, with clinical trials (Birch and Tizard 1967). However, overall the conclusion at this point was that a controlled trial was not justified, as the benefits were clear in many cases treated. In spite of the many unanswered questions there was no doubt that intellectual deterioration could be prevented provided the diet was begun early. The need to take action to diagnose cases soon after birth so treatment could be started at an early age was championed. It became high priority to introduce screening for PKU as soon as possible after birth to enable treatment at the earliest possible age.

By the 1960s scientists and doctors therefore concentrated on developing newborn screening and treatment for early diagnosed cases although it was known that many hundreds of untreated cases with severe mental disabilities were being cared for in mental hospitals. Sadly, it had become clear that there was little that could be done to help late diagnosed individuals, like Sheila, who were already in these institutions.

Development of Newborn Screening for PKU: 1960-1970s

The way in which those with PKU were diagnosed underwent a marked change. Originally, patients were found by screening populations (usually adults) of retarded people in mental institutions. Others, like Sheila, were found by routine testing of mentally retarded infants in special clinics, or by screening the younger siblings of known cases. In the early 1960s, prior to the introduction of universal newborn screening, the role of the family doctor and paediatrician was emphasised by encouraging testing of any baby or infant with signs and symptoms suggestive of PKU such as eczema, failure to thrive, febrile convulsions, slow development, to enable the earliest possible diagnosis and chance of preventing severe brain damage.

In the early stages of newborn screening in the UK, from the late 1950s to mid-1960s, the ferric chloride test for PPA in urine was used. Urine-based methods were used for several years across the UK as there was no suitable blood-based phenylalanine method for newborns at that time. The first programme started in Cardiff in March 1958 using liquid urine collected by mothers when the baby was about three weeks of age (Gibbs and Woolf 1958). The urines were brought to the infant welfare clinic and ferric chloride solution was added. In 1959 a simple paper test strip, marketed as *Phenistix* (Ames Company), became available and was a much easier way to screen rather than collecting liquid urine. The test strip could be simply pressed on a wet nappy and was referred to as the 'nappy' test. It became clear that urine was not a reliable test in the first few weeks of life, as insufficient amounts of PPA are excreted to give a positive test result with ferric chloride. For this reason it was advocated that testing be undertaken a few weeks after birth (Armstrong and Binkley 1956). The City of Birmingham pioneered newborn screening in England using *Phenistix* with testing of all babies born in the city in 1959 at six weeks of age, the same year Sheila was admitted to Chelmsley (Boyd 1961). This study demonstrated that whole population screening of the newborn, undertaken by health visitors in the home, was practicable as a community-based service on this scale, and was the beginning of its introduction on a wider basis. Other locally organised programmes became established and by the early 1960s mass newborn screening using the 'nappy test' was in use or being set up across most of England and Wales (Woolf 1967, Woolf 1968). This was only 10 years after Sheila had been treated. Cases were now being diagnosed early enough for dietary treatment to be effective.

A conference on Phenylketonuria (Medical Research Council 1963), to review the detection and treatment of cases of PKU in the UK, recommended continuation and if possible expansion of the then current screening programmes. The need to collect and share data on detected cases across the country in order to answer some of the outstanding questions about PKU was hi-lighted. This need had been suggested by a group of clinicians in the north of England and was the stimulus to develop a national register of PKU children for the UK in 1963. This was established by the Medical Research Council with Dr F P (Freddie) Hudson at Alder Hey Children's Hospital Liverpool as director. It recorded information on the diagnosis and progress of all patients with PKU in England, Scotland and Wales born on or after 1st Jan 1964; cases from Northern Ireland were included from 1965. The register was maintained by Dr Hudson at Liverpool until his untimely death in 1976 and was then transferred to Great Ormond Street Hospital, London under the administration of Dr Isabel Smith. The establishment of this register was a key development in proving the case for newborn screening and guidance for optimal treatment.

Alongside the work by the MRC, a group of individuals from the north of England formed a new organisation in 1963, the Society for the Study of Inborn Errors of Metabolism (SSIEM) to promote the exchange of ideas between professional workers who are interested in inherited metabolic disorders. The annual symposia of the SSIEM throughout the 1960s became an important forum for discussion and sharing of ideas about PKU and many other metabolic disorders, and rapidly became an international society.

Sadly there were reports of some missed cases and the failure to detect all cases of PKU using a urine-based screening test was becoming clear. The tests using urine were simply not sufficiently reliable. A major breakthrough was the development of a blood-based screening method for phenylalanine by Robert

11. PKU Developments

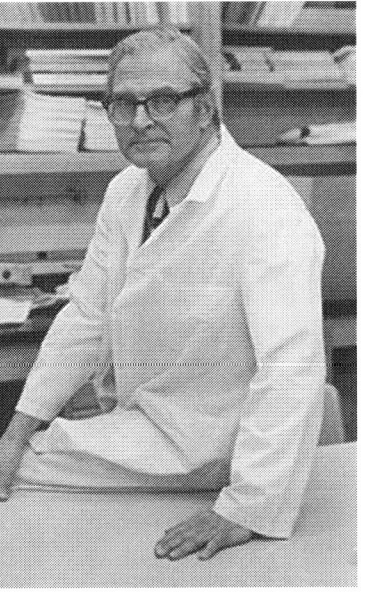
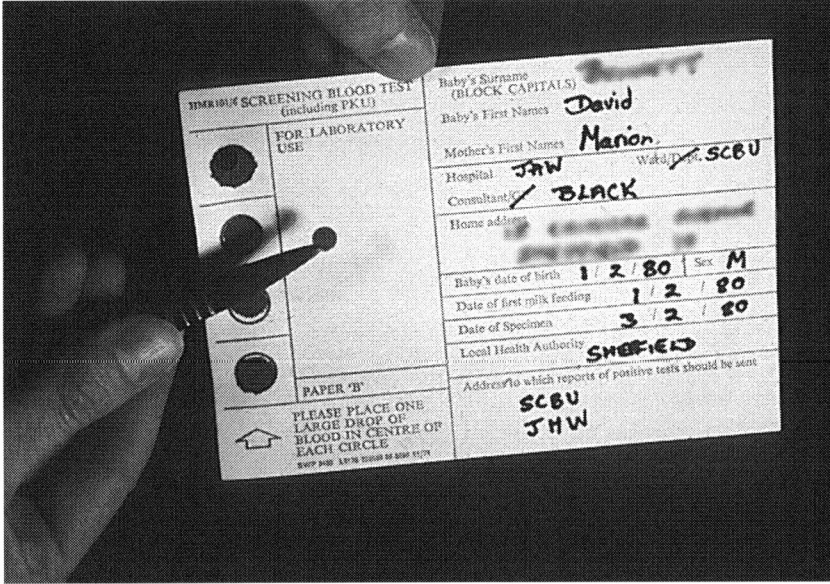

Left: Dr Robert Guthrie in his laboratory c. mid 1980s (photograph courtesy University Archives, State University of New York at Buffalo and kindly provided by The Guthrie family). Right: Blood spot card for newborn screening used in UK c.1980s.

Guthrie in the USA (Guthrie and Susi 1963). Blood was collected on to an absorbent card, dried and a small blood spot punched out. The spot was tested for phenylalanine using a microbiological test and became known worldwide as the 'Guthrie test' or 'heel-prick test', or more recently the blood spot test.

In the early 1960s, mass newborn screening using blood spots began in several of the states of the USA; Scotland started implementation in November 1965 (S.E. Scotland Region Report, 1968). It subsequently became widely established around the world. Alternative blood-based methods to detect phenylalanine were also developed using chromatography or fluorimetry. In the city of Birmingham blood-based newborn screening was introduced by Dr Noel Raine at BCH with a pilot survey in July 1968, and by

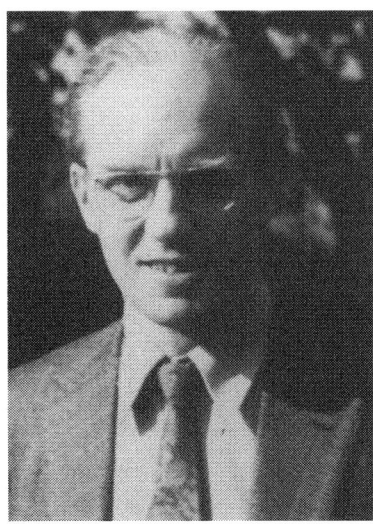

Dr D. Noel Raine Consultant Chemical Pathologist at BCH 1963-1980.

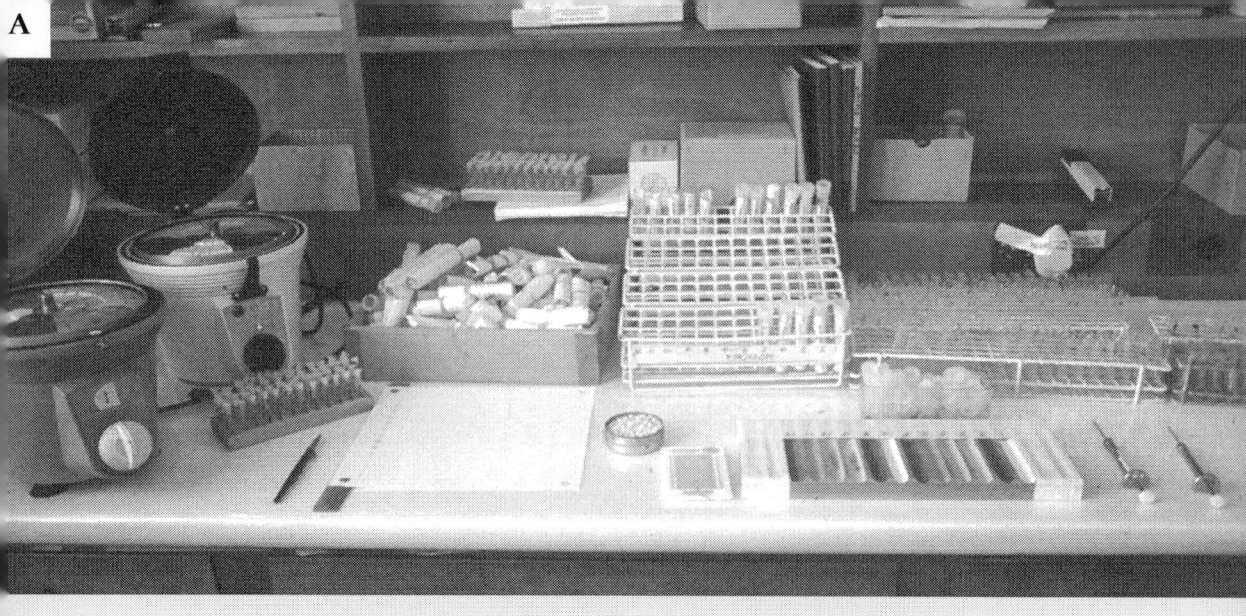

Newborn Screening for PKU at BCH using the 'Scriver' technique 1971 (photographs reproduced courtesy of Nursing Mirror). A. Laboratory Bench. B. The Author receiving specimens. C. Centrifuge for glass capillary tubes. D. Spotting of plasma on to paper. E. Inserting papers into chromatography tank. F. Staining with Ninhydrin. G. Chromatogram showing specimen with increased phenylalanine.

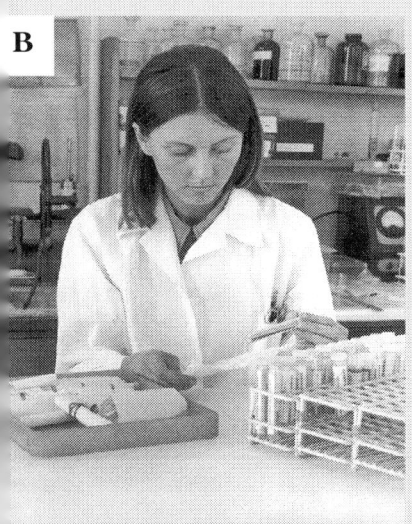
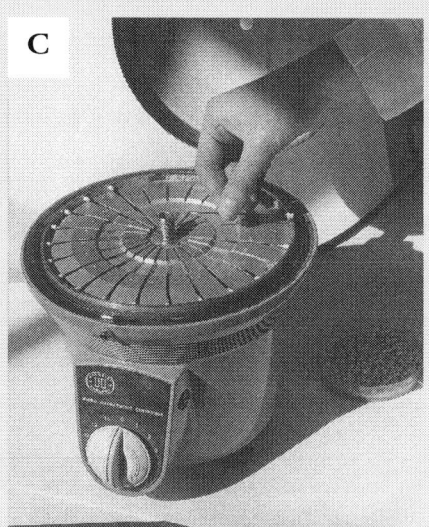
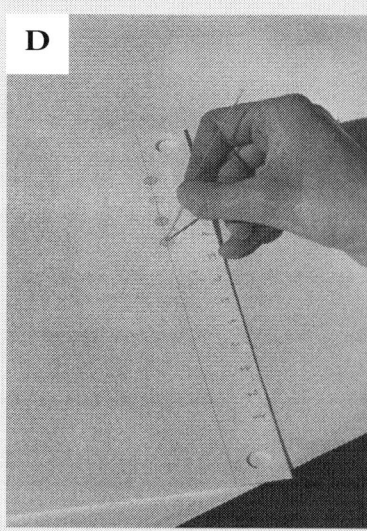
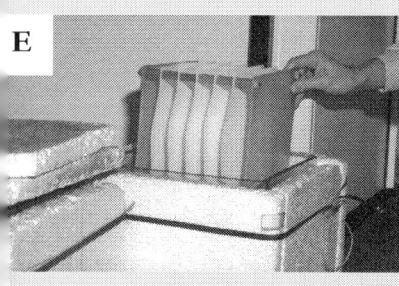
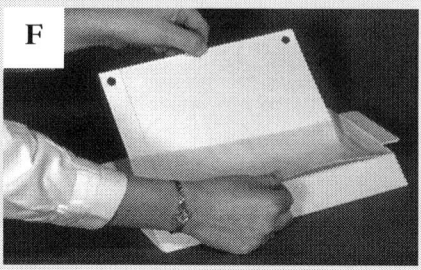
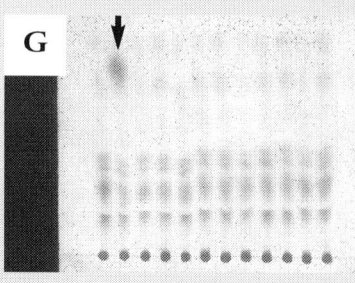

March 1969 all births in the city were included (Mahon 1973). The technique used was paper chromatography for amino acids, devised by Charles Scriver from Canada (Scriver 1964). This was similar to the chromatography method used to diagnose Sheila, albeit with a requirement for only very small blood volumes suitable for newborn babies. Blood was collected in fragile glass capillary tubes and after centrifugation the separated plasma spotted on the paper. As well as PKU a whole range of different disorders could be detected from the resulting amino acid pattern.

An MRC working group was established to assess and compare the different screening tests, and guidelines on screening for England and Wales were issued; these recommended that the Phenistix test should be replaced with a blood test for phenylalanine (DHSS 1967; Welsh Hospital Board 1968). This required heel prick blood collected at 6-14 days of age with services for laboratory testing to be organised on a regional basis. Specimens of either blood spots or liquid blood collected by midwives were sent to centralised laboratories to test for phenylalanine. By 1974 only 1-2% of surviving infants were not being tested for PKU in the neonatal period in the UK, a remarkable achievement. A critical outcome from this work was the demonstration that the IQs of those with PKU, treated from an early age following diagnosis after newborn screening, were similar to those of non PKU age matched controls. The importance of maintaining good control of blood phenylalanine levels was also demonstrated (MRC 1981). Further work by the MRC Working Group produced recommendations on dietary management (MRC 1993).

In 1973 a National Society for PKU for the UK (NSPKU) was founded by two parents to help and support families with PKU, an organisation that has gone from strength to strength. By the mid-1970s, newborn blood spot screening had become routine in most industrialised nations and many other sister organisations of the NSPKU have since been established in other countries. The European Society for Phenylketonuria and Allied Disorders (E.S.PKU) is now an umbrella organisation founded in 1987 comprising about 41 national and regional associations from 31 countries, again established by parents to support families and improve quality of care for those affected. The main event of the E.S.PKU is an annual conference where patients, parents and families, as well as medical and other professionals come together to share experiences and discuss developments and is the venue for the annual Sheila Jones Award (see p.104). International meetings for professionals began to be organised and gave birth to the ISNS in 1991.

Laboratory Assessment of Dietary and Biochemical Control
With the longer term follow up data, from cases diagnosed in the newborn period, scientists began to understand more about how the phenylalanine requirement for growth varied with age and that young babies and infants needed more

phenylalanine in their diets than older children. Several studies were undertaken to investigate the effect of phenylalanine restriction on metabolites (Blainey and Leyton 1963). It became clear that the estimation of PPA in the urine was not a satisfactory measure of dietary control as concentrations became normal (with negative ferric chloride test) at a fairly high phenylalanine level. Similarly urine phenylalanine concentration was not a good measure of control. The importance of monitoring phenylalanine blood levels became appreciated with consequent improvements in laboratory technology, thereby enabling measurement of phenylalanine using smaller sample volumes with greater ease of collection and more rapid turnaround of results.

In the early years it was considered that optimal dietary therapy was best achieved by hospitalisation and so it was normal practice for a newly diagnosed baby to be admitted to hospital for several weeks until the blood phenylalanine levels had stabilised. Plasma phenylalanine measurements were usually carried out every three to seven days whilst in hospital. After discharge the infant would be brought to an outpatients' clinic once or twice every month for blood sampling. In some cases ferric chloride testing on urine was undertaken by the mother at home as a way of checking that the diet was working between blood sampling. These practices continued for many years.

The initial methods of blood/plasma phenylalanine measurement were microbiological and were cumbersome and required large blood volumes. Enzymatic and chromatographic methods became available and allowed blood volumes to be reduced. Further development of blood spot methods in the 1990s reduced the required blood volume even more and enabled greater ease of more frequent measurement.

The UK neonatal screening programme for PKU achieved high coverage and was effective (Smith et al 1991) but there were however still many unanswered questions which continued to occupy scientists:

> What is the optimal value for blood phenylalanine?
> When should blood be taken in relationship to meals?
> When to stop the treatment? – Or could it ever be safely stopped?
> Should all patients detected by newborn screening be treated? – is there a lower limit of blood phenylalanine level before starting treatment?
> Diagnosis of atypical/variant forms of PKU and how to manage these cases?

These were just some of the challenges in the early years post introduction of newborn screening.

12

RECOGNITION OF THE BIRMINGHAM CONTRIBUTION TO PKU TREATMENT

John Gerrard 1962: *'Both Horst and I are in full agreement with Dr Hubble in suggesting Dr Hickmans is worth 50 of us'.*

The John Scott Award
The pioneering work of the team at Birmingham Children's Hospital had not gone unnoticed around the world and although the individuals had gone their separate ways, they were reunited in Birmingham in 1962 to be honoured with a very special award for their work – THE JOHN SCOTT AWARD. This is an international award from the City of Philadelphia to deserving individuals of notable inventions. It is usually given annually and is applicable across a wide range of disciplines.

Who was John Scott?
John Scott born in the 1740s was a pharmacist in Saint Patrick Square in Edinburgh. He is listed as a *'druggist'*, *'apothecary'* or *'chymist'*. He moved to London and died there in 1815. He bequeathed a sum of US $4000 to the City of Philadelphia, the income of which was to be used as an award. Exactly why the award was established in the United States is unclear although John Scott had a long standing interest and connections with the USA and was sympathetic to the ideals of Republicanism. It is felt that the award was a tangible expression of his beliefs. During his life he had numerous contacts in the USA, and friends came over to Edinburgh to study.

In his will he laid down the foundations for the award. Essentially it is an award given to inventors *'whom are particularly deserving because their invention contributed to the comfort, welfare and happiness of human kind'*. It was stated that the award should not exceed a sum of $20 U.S. and would be given with a copper medal inscribed with the words *'To the most deserving'*.

The first John Scott Award was given in 1822 in Philadelphia. From 1822 to 1919 a total of 499 awards were made. They were usually for ideas of limited application rather than fundamental discoveries or inventions. It is a prestigious award not for its financial value but the distinction of its prize winners.

The income from the investment of the fund grew over the years and the individual annual prize was increased to $1,000 from 1920. In 1921 the award became international and wide ranging notably across scientific, medical and engineering disciplines. Prior to 1962 particularly notable award winners include:

1921   Marie Curie: Discovery of Radium
1924   Frederick Banting: Extraction of Pancreatic Insulin
1925   Orville Wright: Development of Flying Machine
1931   Guglielmo Marconi: Wireless Telegraphy
1944   Alexander Fleming: Discovery of Penicillin
1957   Frank Whittle: Invention of Turbo Jet engine

The John Scott Award 1962
In 1962 Dr Hickmans, Professor Bickel and Professor Gerrard were given this prestigious award for their work on the preparation of the diet for PKU in Birmingham in 1951. As for all previous awards it included a monetary sum (winners each received US $333.33), a certificate and a large copper medal *'TO THE MOST DESERVING'* for each of them.

The original letter to Professor Gerrard from the City of Philadelphia notifying him of the award, and congratulatory letters to Dr Hickmans from the University of Birmingham, the Children's Hospital and the United Birmingham Hospitals are reproduced in Appendix V.

At the time of the award Dr Hickmans was retired and living in Wolverhampton. Horst Bickel was Professor of Paediatrics at Marburg University, Germany and John

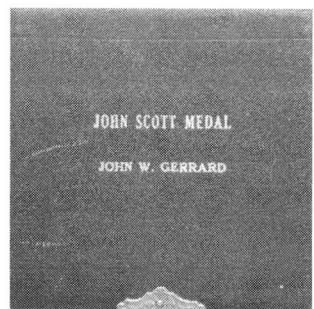 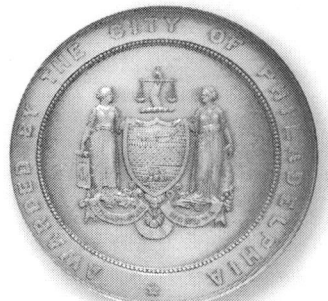 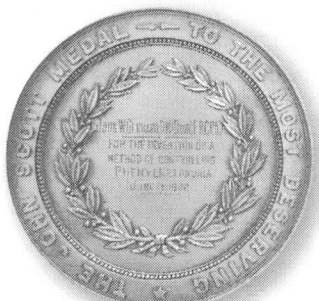

The John Scott Medal presented to Professor John Gerrard (photographs kindly provided by the Gerrard Family).

12. Recognition of the Birmingham Contribution to PKU Treatment

Gerrard was Professor of Paediatrics at the University of Saskatchewan, Canada. On 24th October 1962 an event hosted by the Medical Faculty of the University of Birmingham and the Midland Region of the Association of Clinical Biochemists (ACB) took place at Birmingham Children's Hospital to present the award. Initially there was some doubt about whether all three award winners would be able to attend but this did occur. Evelyn Hickmans, John Gerrard with his wife Betty, his parents and an aunt and uncle, and Horst Bickel with his wife Stella, all attended.

The ceremony for presenting the award was organised by the Midland Region of the ACB, as part of their 78th scientific meeting, at the Children's Hospital.

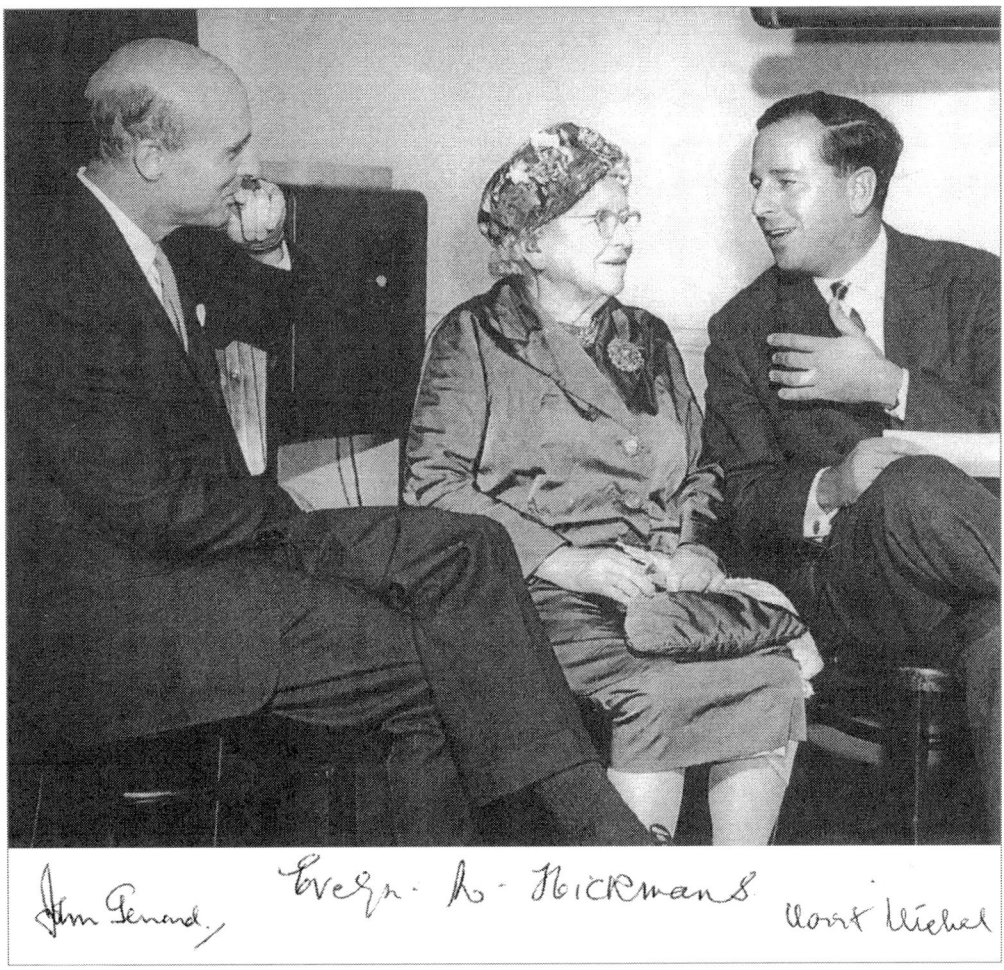

The occasion of the John Scott Award at Birmingham Children's Hospital 1962 (photograph kindly provided by the Gerrard Family).

Letters concerning the meeting are shown in Appendix V. Dr Neville Belton, an ACB member, and a PhD student in Medical Biochemistry at Birmingham University at the time, recalls this special event. It was attended by over 60 distinguished guests – the signature list of many of those is reproduced in Appendix V. The meeting commenced with tea, priced 1/6d (8 pence) and was followed by the presentation of the award. It had been planned that the US Ambassador in London would be presenting the award but in fact it was Dr W. Greulich, Scientific Attaché to the US Embassy in London who came. The presentation was followed by a lecture on 'QUANTITATIVE PAPER CHROMATOGRAPHY IN BIO-CHEMICAL INVESTIGATIONS' by Professor IE Bush, Professor of Physiology, University of Birmingham (BCH Archive).

It is of interest that 24th October was the height of the Cuban Missile Crisis for the USA and almost certainly this was the reason the Ambassador himself did not attend the award ceremony in person. An extract from Wikipedia for 24th October 1962 shows the severity of the situation: *'The crisis was continuing unabated, and in the evening of October 24, the Soviet news agency TASS broadcast a telegram from Khrushchev to Kennedy in which Khrushchev warned that the United States' "outright piracy" would lead to war'*.

Before presenting the award Dr Greulich stated that: *'more than 10,000 adults suffering from PKU were in mental institutions in Britain and the United States, most of them with a mental age of under 3 years'* (Ann Clin Biochem 1963). It was a stark statement about the severity of the disorder if individuals went untreated and reminded us of how things would have continued without the development of the diet. Dr Greulich went on to say: *'They developed a special diet, which if started within a few days after birth, will permit full mental development of those children. The invention of this diet was involved and complex but is now extensively used in both countries and elsewhere with success'* (Birmingham Post 1962).

The scientific meeting was followed by a reception and dinner, price 27/6d (£1.38p) at Staff House at the University, hosted by Birmingham Medical School and the ACB (see Appendix V). Professor Hubble (Professor of Paediatrics at BCH) gave a toast to the guests; the response by Professor Gerrard on behalf of himself, Professor Bickel and Dr Hickmans is reproduced in Appendix V. In the speech it was mentioned that, sadly, they had not heard anything about the fate of Sheila or Mrs Jones:

'We have not heard I am sorry to say, from Mrs Jones, the mother of the original Phenylketonuric, Sheila for she has had a nervous breakdown and both she and her daughter are now in institutions. The doctor, Dr Allin, who originally referred Sheila to us, is still in practice here in Birmingham, but I am sorry to say that it was only yesterday that he was first made aware of the chain of events which he set in motion

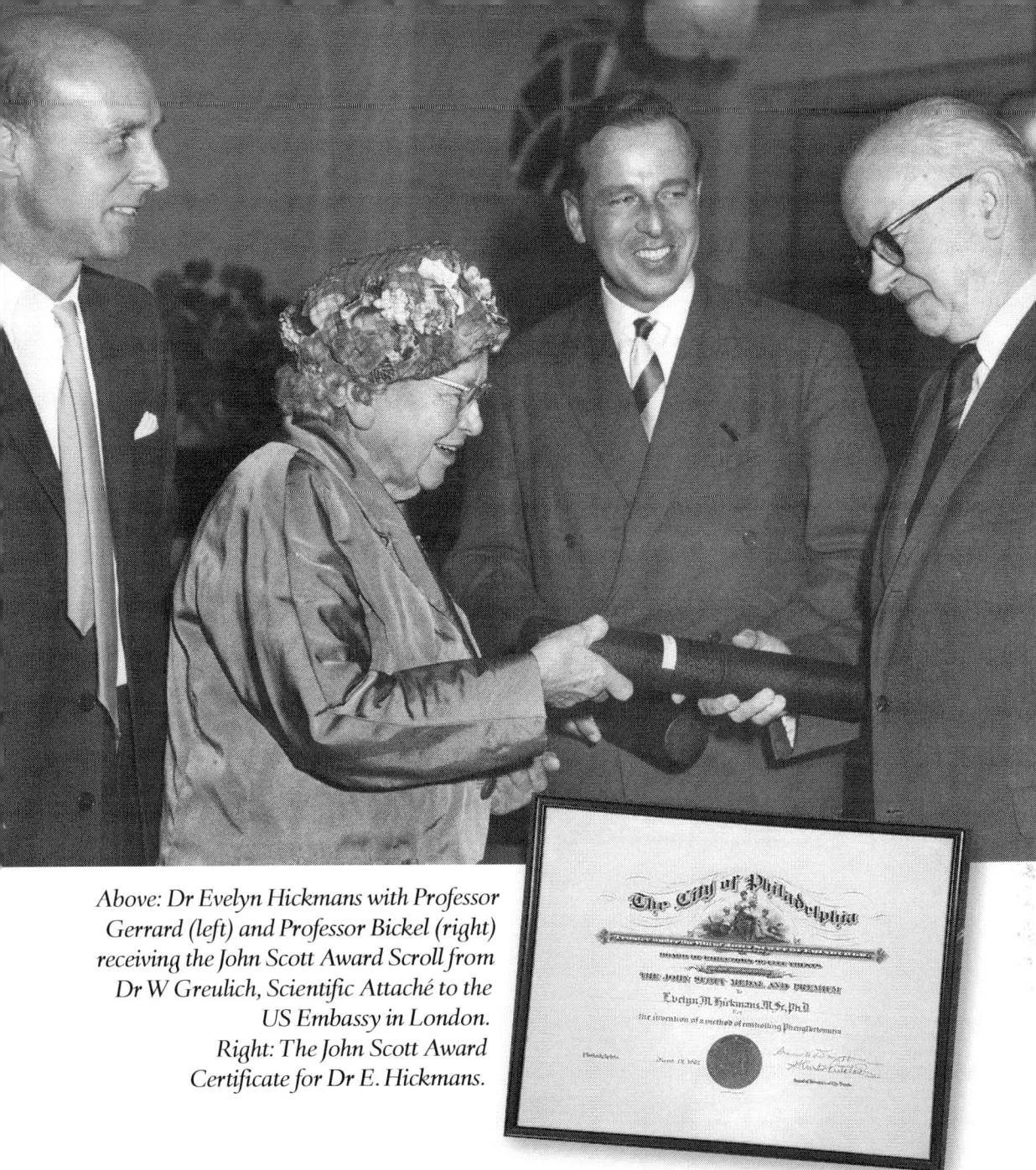

Above: Dr Evelyn Hickmans with Professor Gerrard (left) and Professor Bickel (right) receiving the John Scott Award Scroll from Dr W Greulich, Scientific Attaché to the US Embassy in London.
Right: The John Scott Award Certificate for Dr E. Hickmans.

when he asked Mrs Jones to bring Sheila to see us over 11 years ago and he is still unaware of the fact that she was a phenylketonuric, nor does he realise what the disease phenylketonuria means'.

Clearly it had been wrongly assumed that Mary Jones' brief periods in a psychiatric hospital for treatment had become long term.

The giving of this award places the achievements of all three professionals in the international arena. In his speech, Professor Gerrard paid particular tribute to Evelyn Hickmans and emphasized that although the preparation of the phenylalanine free formula is now carried out commercially *'it was no mean achievement'*. He went on to say: *'The present occasion however affords more than local recognition, for the award, particularly as it comes from another country, ensures a niche for her in the international field, and as long as there are Phenylketonurics to be treated, the name of Dr Hickmans will be coupled with their care and management'*.

Reflecting in 2019 about how all this came about, culminating in the John Scott Award, the words of Jon Gerrard, son of Professor John W Gerrard are particularly pertinent:

'One of the fascinating aspects of the work undertaken was that only a few years before, Horst Bickel and John Gerrard were both serving as doctors in World War II but on opposite sides – Dr Gerrard was in the First Reconnaissance Regiment for England and Horst Bickel in the navy for Germany. It was an extraordinary demonstration of how these two individuals were able to collaborate together so soon after the war to make such a major advance in helping children with PKU. This may have been possible because John Gerrard had spent some time in Germany before the war and had become friends with Germans of his own age. This plus the fact that Stella and John Gerrard's wife were friends may have also helped enable the two of them, together with Evelyn Hickmans, to work together to achieve what none of them could have achieved alone' (personal communication Jon Gerrard 2019).

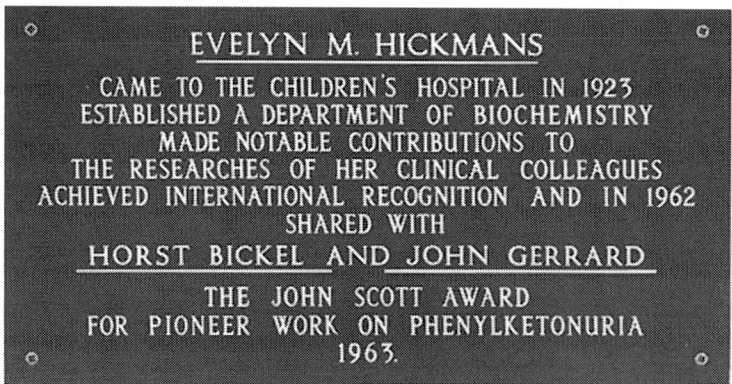

The John Scott Award – Commemorative plaque.

The event to celebrate this work and the giving of the award at BCH was commemorated with a special plaque in Clinical Chemistry, initially located at the Ladywood site and since re-located to the current Children's Hospital (Clinical Chemistry) at the city centre site on Steelhouse Lane.

12. Recognition of the Birmingham Contribution to PKU Treatment

The 25th Anniversary Meeting of the John Scott Award – 1987

On 24th October 1987, a special celebratory meeting of the John Scott Award took place at BCH, 25 years to the day since the original award ceremony. Professor Gerrard with his wife Betty from Saskatoon, Professor Bickel from Germany and Dr Brian Rudd from Birmingham were able to attend together with over 100 delegates to celebrate the giving of the award 25 years earlier and the progress made since their original work; Dr Hickmans had sadly died in 1972. Tom Day whose role as a young student in 1951/2 had not previously been fully appreciated also attended. It was a very special occasion for the individuals who had played such an important role in the history of PKU and for those who had subsequently worked in biochemistry at BCH to be able to return to the hospital to celebrate the award with a scientific meeting and a celebratory dinner at Birmingham Botanical Gardens (Appendix V).

The author wishes to acknowledge help from the late Stuart Mann (former Principal Scientist and Business Manager at BCH) for undertaking the photography below.

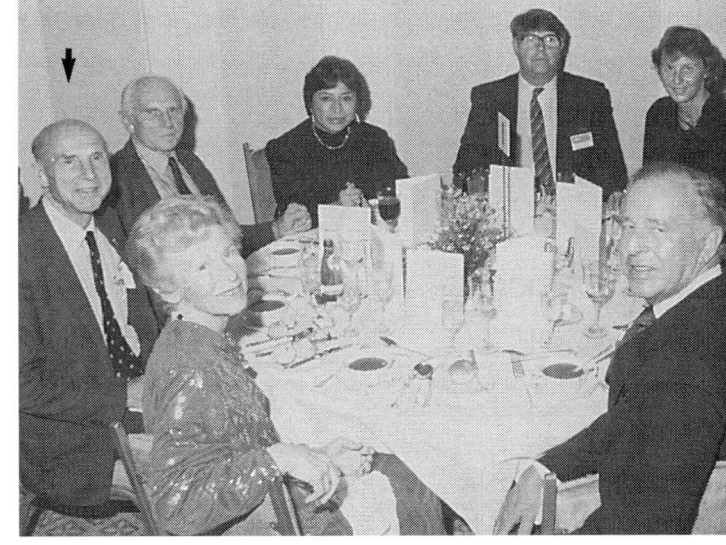

Right: Jubilee Dinner 1987 at Birmingham Botanical Gardens (from arrow anticlockwise): Professor John Gerrard, Mrs Betty Gerrard, Professor Horst Bickel, Dr Anne Green, Dr John Lines, Mrs Lines, Dr Ben Wood.
Bottom left: Professor Horst Bickel (left) and Professor John Gerrard (right).
Bottom right: Professor John Gerrard (left) and Dr Brian Rudd (right).

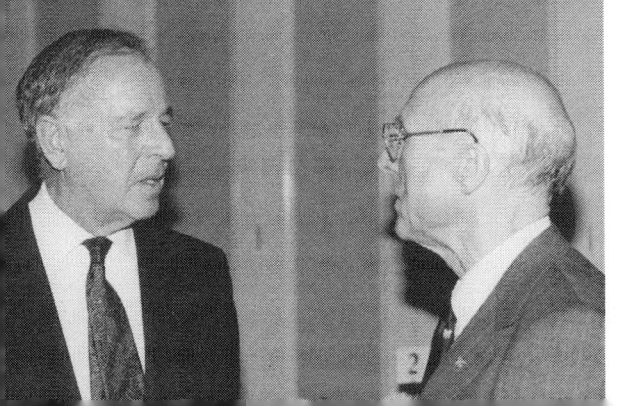
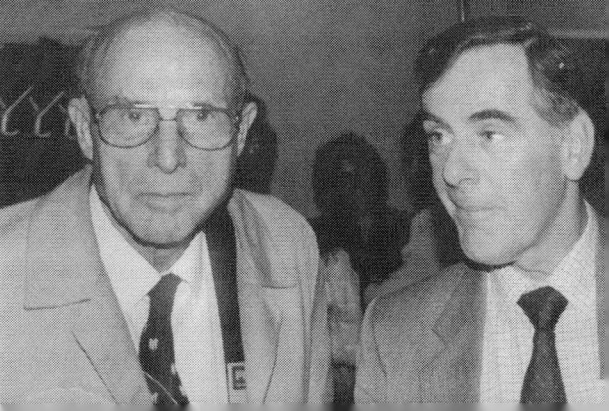

The Sheila Jones Award 2018
The recognition of the importance of this pioneering work by Drs Bickel, Gerrard and Hickmans does not just belong to the professionals. The contribution by Sheila, and in particular her mother Mary, to the world of PKU was the stimulus to develop a specific award for advocacy.

In 2017 the E.S.PKU together with the Birmingham Children's Hospital, and with permission from the Jones family, established the Sheila Jones Award. This prestigious award is for advocacy work and is given to a volunteer, a patient or family member who has demonstrated courage, innovation, hard work, commitment and tenacity and made a real difference to the lives of others with PKU. This is the first public recognition given to supporters of patients who have done amazing things for the PKU community.

The first award in 2018 was presented to Laura Petreus, a mother from Baia Mare, Romania. Laura has two children with PKU and has single-handedly done so much to further the cause for PKU in her country. She has worked hard and campaigned tirelessly over many years with determination and courage very much in the spirit of Mary Jones. She was a most worthy winner of this first award. In Laura's words (Muresan, 2018): *'This award carries the suffering of all children diagnosed late with PKU and all the joy of early detection by neonatal screening, who have been treated correctly. I will continue to fight for PKU'.*

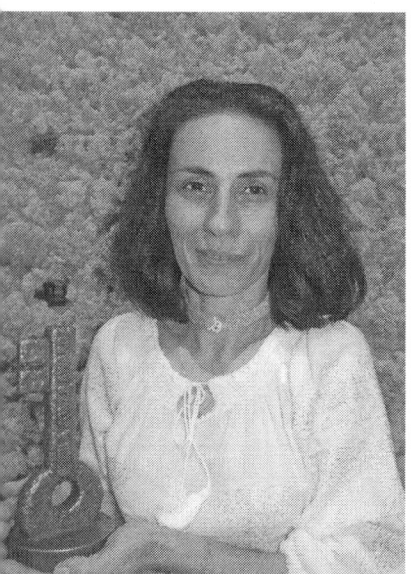 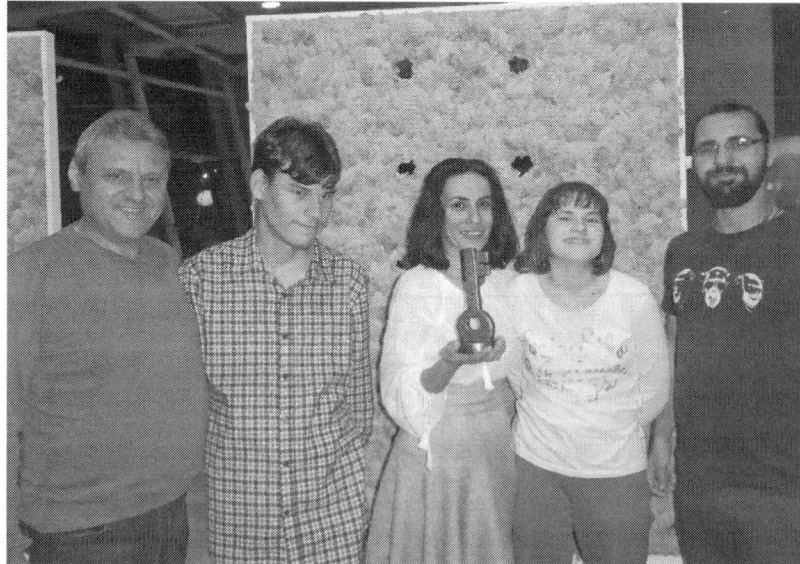

Left: Laura Petreus – winner of the first Sheila Jones Award 2018. Right: Laura Petreus and family (photographs reproduced with kind permission of Laura Petreus).

12. Recognition of the Birmingham Contribution to PKU Treatment

The award was given at the annual E.S.PKU conference in Venice, November 2018 where over 500 delegates attended, of whom about 120 had PKU. The award itself takes the form of a key and is a reminder of the keys which Horst Bickel used to get Sheila's attention in his film. The key is symbolic of 'opening the door to treatment' and a key to the future of PKU.

The award is to recognise the legacy of Sheila Jones and is a fitting tribute to Sheila, Mary and the Jones family. It will be an annual event for the E.S.PKU.

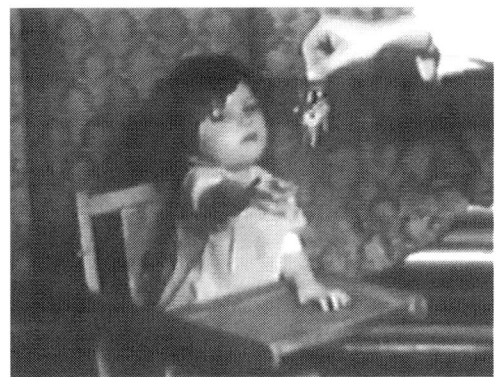

Sheila reaching for Dr Bickel's keys 1952 (photograph reproduced with kind permission of the Jones Family).

13

REFLECTIONS 2019

Dr Ashok Roy, Brooklands Hospital 2019: *'A reminder of the potential benefits of science but also the price paid of being a pioneer'.*

Phenylketonuria Today
What about PKU today? The disorder is part of the newborn screening programme for the UK and most developed countries across the world. The early developments in the UK led the world and were largely due to the enthusiasm and dedication of several early pioneers, including Freddie Hudson, Joe Ireland, Louis Woolf, Noel Raine and George Komrower. Not only did PKU screening extend across the world but it also provided the infrastructure for screening for other disorders. Newborn screening continues to expand geographically as does the number of disorders now screened for, albeit there are huge differences between countries. This is sometimes because of specific issues for a particular population or a more cautious/proactive approach to screening. In the UK nine disorders are currently tested for using tandem mass spectrometry technology on blood spot samples taken on day five of age. The pace of expansion to include other disorders has been greatest in the USA.

Diagnosis of PKU cases in 2018/9 for the West Midlands region of England (BCH Laboratory) and the UK

	Total Babies screened	PKU cases
West Midlands*	67452	7 (total 177 cases since 1983) (average 5 cases diagnosed per year)
UK**	736010	87 (total 590 cases since 2011) (average 74 cases diagnosed per year)

Sources: *West Midlands Newborn Screening Laboratory (Preece and Goddard 2019) and the **NHS Newborn Blood Spot Screening Programme (PHE 2019) with special thanks to Dr Philippa Goddard*, Mary Anne Preece* and Christine Cavanagh**.

13. Reflections 2019

The effectiveness of the screening programme is impressive with 97.8% babies screened ≤17 days of age in England. This has been made possible with the use of IT linking the programme to the birth notification system. This idea was pioneered by Noel Raine, again at BCH, and was in place by the mid-1980s (Griffiths 1987); there are now national systems across England and Wales. The UK programme achieves early treatment for most babies with referral to a clinical team for start of treatment by 14 days of age. This prompt start of treatment has led to excellent outcomes for those with PKU who are now able to have normal lives and achieve their ambitions.

The success of treatment has been possible partly because of the improvements and availability of dietary products. Protein substitutes have been developed beyond all recognition since the early mixtures produced in the 1950s. Some of those produced commercially in 2019 are illustrated below.

Improvements in dietary management have likewise been huge (MacDonald 2016). There is now guidance on age at start of treatment, optimal blood phenylalanine levels at different ages, timing of blood sampling and continuation of diet for life. Multidisciplinary teams now help the patient and family and include clinical psychologists and support/liaison workers with greater use of patient advocates. The role of parents and families in the development of products has been of great benefit. Collaboration with community services has led to the greater involvement of health professionals in the home and home delivery of dietary products.

Use of digital technology has had a great impact on communication and for educational purposes. Patient educational websites, clinical health records, personal health records, patient apps for storage of dietary information and to assist with self-management of diet, patient webinars and electronic messaging of blood results are examples of its use. Social media is used widely for patient education and communication and allows patients/families to support each other.

With the growing numbers of patients in clinics, and continuation of diet, provision of adult PKU services has been a major development with transition of

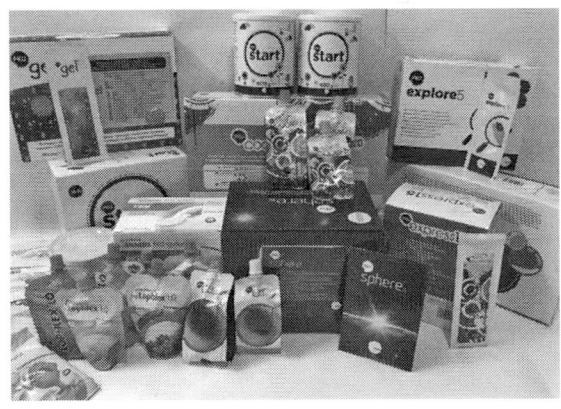

PKU Protein substitute products 2019 (photograph kindly provided by Alex Pinto and Professor Anita MacDonald, Dietetics, BCH).

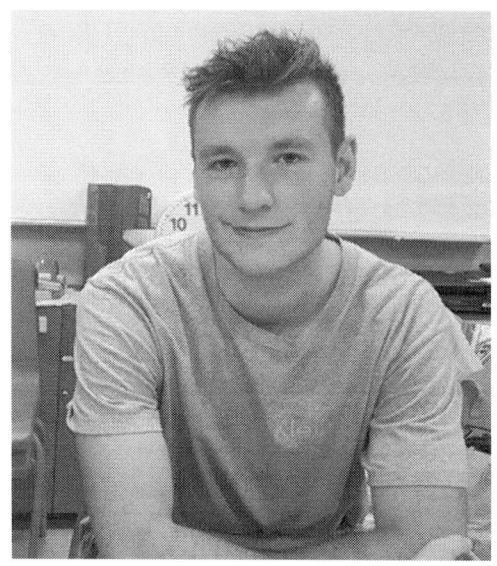 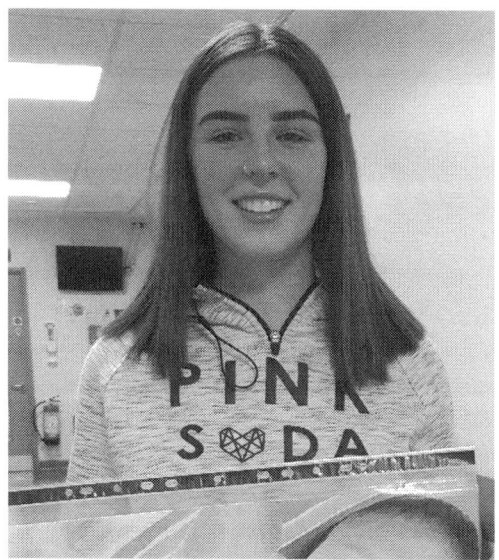

Successfully treated PKU Patients at BCH:
left: Cameron – A Medical Student, right: Taila – A Theatre Art Student
(photographs courtesy of Professor Anita MacDonald, Dietetics, BCH).

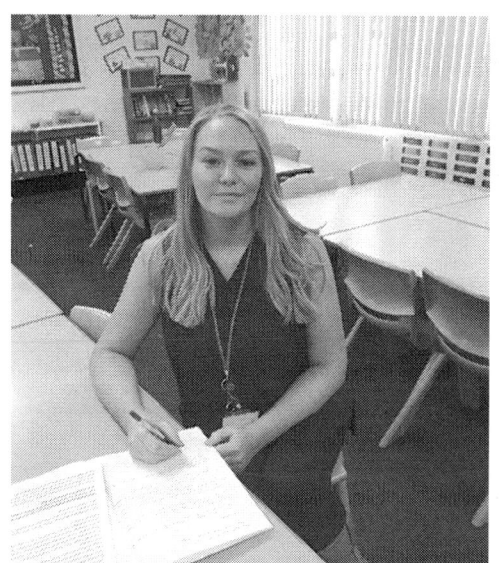 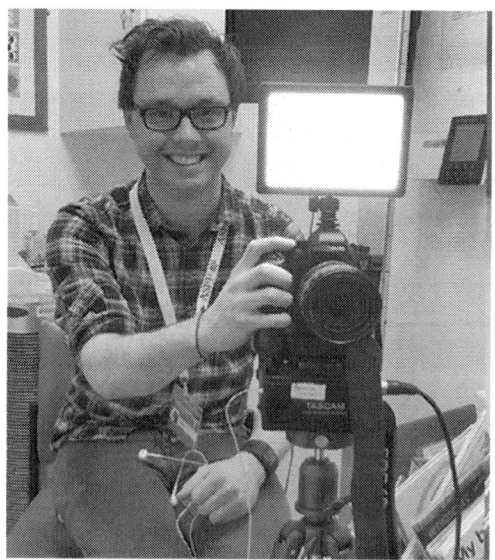

Successfully treated PKU Patients at BCH:
left: Louise – A Teacher, right: Tom – A Film Maker and University Lecturer.
(photographs courtesy of Professor Anita MacDonald, Dietetics, BCH).

patients between paediatric and adult teams. The principle of diet for life has become widely accepted. However, we must not forget that in spite of all the advances, the diet is restrictive and for some tough to adhere to, requiring determination and dedication. The overwhelming result however is that we can now expect PKU persons to achieve as these young adults (see opposite) have from the West Midlands. There are numerous inspirational stories – these are just an example.

As well as the improvements in services there have also been great advances in the understanding of PKU at the molecular level. The human phenylalanine hydroxylase gene was isolated and cloned (Woo 1983) and opened the way for further important research and developments. There is now recognition of over 950 variant forms (gene mutations) of the disease (Blau 2016) giving rise to a continuous spectrum of the disease ranging from mild forms requiring no intervention to the most severe. Most individuals with PKU have two different mutations (compound heterozygotes). Sheila had two different mutations each known to result in total loss of enzyme activity hence explaining the severity of her presentation. Although this understanding of the molecular basis of the disorder brought about the possibility of pre-natal diagnosis, there has been virtually no demand for routine genetic testing in clinical practice since knowing the specific variant (genotype) is currently not thought to be useful in guiding dietary management for PKU.

This understanding of the molecular basis of PKU and the ability to characterize the severity of the disorder can help predict whether new treatment possibilities, such as with the cofactor tetrahydrobiopterin, might be of benefit. Tetrahydrobiopterin can be used to enhance any residual phenylalanine hydroxylase activity (see figure on p.23). In 2008 the first pharmacological therapy for PKU was licenced in Europe, sapropterin dihydrochloride (Kuvan®, BioMarin, CA, USA), a synthetic form of tetrahydrobiopterin. It is only effective in a subset of patients (around 20 to 30%) mainly those with mild or moderate PKU. It lowers blood phenylalanine concentrations and improves phenylalanine tolerance thus allowing a greater intake of dietary phenylalanine. It is either given orally with a relaxed low phenylalanine diet or it may replace diet therapy completely, depending on the individual's response to the drug (Muntau 2018).

Other forms of treatment to reduce the phenylalanine load in the body are possibilities for some patients. These include phenylalanine ammonium lyase (PAL), an enzyme which converts phenylalanine into low concentrations of ammonia and a non-toxic by-product, trans-cinnamic acid. In May 2019 the European Medicines Agency granted marketing authorization for Pegvaliase, a derivative of PAL (trade name Palynziq®), for adult PKU patients with poor control. This product substantially lowers blood phenylalanine levels, thus enabling an increased dietary protein intake. There are however reported side effects including injection site reactions, anaphylactic episodes and joint pain (Longo et al 2019). It may be an option for patients who cannot achieve adequate blood phenylalanine levels with diet alone.

For the future there are other new emerging treatments including gene therapy (Lichter-Konecki 2019) and genetically modified bacteria which metabolise phenylalanine (Isabella et al 2018). The first clinical trials with gene therapy are expected to start in 2020.

With the advances in treatment new questions have emerged to continue to challenge clinicians and scientists for the future:

> Are there any better biomarkers than phenylalanine to monitor treatment?
> Adequacy of patient follow up – how many patients are lost to follow up?
> What co-morbidities might be associated with PKU for those early patients who are now approaching 50 years of age and more, since start of treatment?
> What is the impact on mental health for those with treated PKU – particularly incidence of anxiety/depression?
> What are the issues for the provision of care for the elderly who have PKU?

With these important questions in mind, whatever answers emerge with time, we must not forget Sheila's story and the many others with PKU diagnosed in the early years who could not benefit from treatment and suffered the severe consequences of the effects of the untreated disorder.

As we reflect on the huge advances and go back to where it started for Sheila in 1951, we can conclude that PKU is a particularly good example where manipulation of a biochemical pathway can reduce or prevent the harmful effects of the disorder and is an example which has also been subsequently successfully applied to many other disorders. The discovery of a method of effectively treating PKU radically altered attitudes towards the possibilities of benefitting at least some individuals with mental handicap. Until then it was assumed that such cases could not be treated and PKU had a very gloomy prognosis. PKU has led the way for many other disorders especially with regard to demonstrating the benefits derived from a large scale screening programme. Who could have imagined just how far things have developed in less than a lifetime. It is particularly pertinent to end these with a quote from Professor John Squire, University of Birmingham from over 50 years ago at the time of the John Scott Award 1962 (Appendix IV, set 3):

13. Reflections 2019

'Ultimately perhaps, when the true nature of many more specific defects underlying mental disorders becomes sufficiently understood, this will turn out to be the most important result (our attitude of benefitting a proportion of mentally handicapped children) of these researchers conducted 10 years ago at Birmingham Children's Hospital'.

Sheila's Life – from her Brothers

'Mum kept us together'.

When writing this book no one has been able to speak with either Sheila or Mary about their lives. However throughout this story Sheila had four brothers. Mary had two sons before Sheila, Terry born 14th February 1945 and Trevor born 7th July 1948, and later had two further sons Philip born 6th November 1954 and William (Liam) born 29th June 1959. Sheila and Trevor were biological siblings. In spite of their adverse living circumstances much of the time in poverty, particularly at Aston, and the fact that they had no father around the home, Sheila and her brothers were brought up as a close knit and loving family by Mary. She fiercely defended them at all times. What do Sheila's brothers recall about their sister, their Mum and the family life?

In 2016, Sheila's brothers knew very little about her medical condition and had at that time not fully appreciated the significance of the contribution which had been made to the world of PKU by their family. They had only begun to learn about PKU as a condition when it became a topic of discussion in Trevor's extended family. They now reflect on their lives and those of their mother and sister in the knowledge of what has been achieved. This has helped them understand and come to terms with what is a sad story for their sister and an exceptionally hard life for their mother. They had never had things fully explained and Trevor admits he had been scared of having children of his own in case they were *'like Sheila'*.

The two elder brothers were close in age to Sheila and lived with her until she was admitted to Chelmsley. Although they have few detailed recollections of Sheila at an early age they did know that all was not right. The question asked in the family was: *'do you think she will ever get better?'* They puzzled as to how all this had started and concluded: *'Mum must have taken Sheila to Dr Allin our family doctor on Fox Hollies Road'. 'Mum must have been worried about Sheila'.* They remember the names of Dr Bickel and Dr Gerrard being mentioned by their Mum and the numerous visits she made with Sheila to the Children's Hospital. This dominated the family life over many years and reduced the amount of time Mary had for bringing up and helping her boys. Terry remembers being taken on trips to the Children's Hospital on the bus and sitting in the waiting room whilst his Mum and Sheila went in to see the doctors and had blood taken. He wondered what was going on – he was only six years old.

Terry and Trevor remember Sheila being on a special diet at home and have vivid memories of Sheila being fed *'stuff from a big black jar which Mum collected from the hospital – Mum had to hold her down and spoon it in'*. They remember Sheila struggling; they describe the stuff as like a *'tar'*. *'Our Mum had to do this for quite a few years'*. The special diet mix was later in a round blue tin – *'it was white powdery stuff – Mum used to make it up with water'*. They recall Sheila crying and struggling when Mary was giving her the diet, *'our Mum had to force feed her twice a day'*. They reflect on how Mary would have gone to the hospital every week with Sheila to collect the diet and bring it back on the bus. *'We were poor and our Mum would have needed a bus fare. Bringing the diet home would have been heavy – a carrier bag job'*. They don't recall much about what Sheila had to eat in the early days other than this terrible mixture. As Sheila got older and presumably was no longer on the strict diet they vividly describe how she loved, as a special treat, hard boiled eggs, chopped up and mixed with butter in a cup – *'she couldn't get enough! Also tea! – by the gallons'*.

They have stories about Sheila's difficult behaviour and how disruptive she was in the home; Mary had to watch over her all the time. *'We weren't taking much notice about what was going on – we were only young kids and we just let Mum get on with it'*. They didn't see much improvement in Sheila's behaviour but do remember her hair changing colour from fair to dark. *'Sheila had blonde mousey coloured hair, not like the dark colour on the photograph'*. This had been a puzzle to them.

They can remember Sheila still sitting in a pram when she was quite a big girl and they used to take her out on their own in the pram to a local park with memories of being stared at by passers-by – *'**they** must be thinking "what is a big girl like that doing in a pram?" – **they** didn't know she couldn't stand or walk at that time. I was that embarrassed as **they** used to stare and I would shout at them as my way of coping'*. When Sheila was older and started to walk she never wore shoes and always walked on her tip toes; this was a feature which continued throughout her life. The nursing staff at Chelmsley think she may have had some surgery to try and correct this but the problem remained and she had to have special shoes made.

There was a sadness from the brothers when confirming that Sheila never spoke a single word and there were very few times when she would engage in play or other normal childhood activities. An incident with chewing gum sticks in Trevor's mind: Sheila was sat on the floor in front of the fire in the back-to-back house – he stuck a piece of chewing gum on the fireguard and as it melted it began to move down the fireguard. *'Sheila got very excited and she wanted me to make it happen again, for me to feel I got a response was great; there were very few times you got a reaction from her'*.

13. Reflections 2019

Terry and Trevor were very aware that their Mum had mental health issues and the local authorities became involved with the family during the mid-late 1950s. *'We sometimes got into trouble – not sure why as we were not particularly boisterous kids – we were well behaved really and didn't cause any bother but, I remember on one occasion drawing on the wallpaper with lipstick and getting told off by some official – I got a real telling off.* Trevor: *'**They** used to frighten me to death! I can remember the two of us going to get coal out the back with a buggy and I found a 10 'bob' (shilling) note – I gave it to Mum when **they** weren't looking'.*

Mary didn't have a lot of time to spend with her two eldest sons as she was so busy looking after Sheila during the time of the dietary treatment in the early-mid 1950s, and undoubtedly they suffered because of this. *'Our Mum had to look after Sheila 24 hours a day and had so much on her mind about Sheila that we got swept to one side'.* They missed out on help with schooling especially learning to read and write – *'I feel I was held back'.* The brothers reflect on how it affected them growing up especially the various times they were taken to Children's Homes by Social Services – *'we went to Father Hudson's at Coleshill whilst Mum was in hospital to give her a bit of a rest'.* They had no family to look after them – *'We had no dad, no cousins, no aunts and uncles or grandad, we had nobody. Our Mum really had it hard'.*

Terry and Trevor really had no idea what was going on with Sheila. *'I thought she had an illness and would get better. After all the powders and stuff that was brought in for her diet I thought she would be alright in the end'.* Mary never explained anything to them and they describe their Mum as *'secretive'* who didn't share things, even when they were older, about what was going on with Sheila. Maybe Mary didn't know what to say to them, how to explain it all and didn't know what Sheila's future would be like. *'She kept everything to herself'.* They admit they didn't ask their Mum very much – *'didn't seem important at the time'.*

Dr Bickel has described how Mary was insistent that Sheila should have some treatment and that it was her persistence that persuaded him and his colleagues to go about preparation of the diet. This has surprised Sheila's brothers as they did not see 'their Mum' as being assertive. *'If you knew Mum she wouldn't say boo to a goose. She wouldn't speak up about things – the only time I remember her speaking up was when someone hit me'.* On further thinking about it they only saw that side of Mary when she was needing to stand up for her children and conclude with a sense of pride *'our Mum was forceful to get the diet for Sheila's treatment'.*

They reflect now about what was going on during all those years for their Mother *'Mum must have had it hard, looking after Sheila 24 hours a day. I remember that she took in lodgers and had a lot of different part time jobs'* – all this was to try to make ends meet and provide for the family. They knew how important Sheila was to Mary – her regular visits to Chelmsley for over 20 years, taking Sheila her favourite things and the single photograph of her on the living room wall at Aston. There were no other photos as the family didn't have a camera. *'We were poor'.*

All the effort and anguish for Mary coping with everything on her own in extreme poverty undoubtedly was the catalyst for her own health problems. In the words of Sheila's brothers: *'It broke Mum'*. However Mary was strong and fiercely protective of the family and determined to keep the Jones children together at all costs. This has come through loud and clear throughout the whole story. *'She could just have let us all go in a home – but she didn't. She kept us together'.*

The traumatic move to Aston was a particularly difficult time and one which even now they can't understand how it came about – it had a huge impact on them. They go over and over in their minds; *'Why did they move? How had it been allowed?'* In spite of all the difficulties living in a back-to-back house they clearly had lots of fun times and in other ways fondly remember their time at Aston playing with the other children in the communal yard – *'there was about 30 kids up the yard. We were a happy family – as kids we didn't see the problems – it was a great community in Aston – in many ways it was the best times. We had nothing but everyone had nothing'*. They recount the story of one occasion when the ragman came round the backs – they took a dress of Mary's (unknown to their Mum) and swopped it for a live chicken! The chicken was running around the living room and Sheila went hysterical when she saw it, grabbed it and threw it on the fire! Worried about what Mary would say the boys rushed out and begged the ragman to give them the dress back which he did. By now, towards the end of the time living at Aston, Sheila was a strong girl with a mind of her own and would sometimes take herself off and wander about.

Inner city post-war poverty continued and the welfare state provision in the community was very limited. Whilst living in Aston around 1959-1960 there was the beginnings of more organised social support for the family. Trevor: *'a little bit to help our Mum. The Family Services Unit were a godsend. They helped our Mum with clothes, furniture and nick-nacks and other things for the house. Sometimes they would take us all out on day trips. They would also give us presents at Christmas – a bag of marbles. Every now and then some people from the Sacred Heart Church would visit our Mum – two or three times a year and sometimes give our Mum a little brown envelope – I think it was money from the church. It was usually around Christmas time'*. The need to provide for her family was always evident – Trevor recalls that his wedding present from his Mum was a bag of sugar and slices of bacon!

'We all knew Sheila was at Chelmsley – Mum went all the time to see her. Mum said she was in hospital. She went every month to visit for about one to two hours and would take Sheila her favourite things'. Mary would make a flask of tea at home to take with biscuits for Sheila and a volunteer from the FSU would take Mary by car. *'It was a long way with no public transport and a big thing for her to make the*

13. Reflections 2019

visit'. Trevor describes how the family link worker, Dorothy, even after she had retired, continued to come in her car to take Mary to visit Sheila. *'Dorothy never really retired and continued to make sure that someone would come to our house to take our Mum to see Sheila. Sheila would drink her tea and then run off after a few minutes. When Mum got back I used to ask her "how's Sheila?" Mum didn't say much. I think we all knew how bad she was and she couldn't be at home'.*

On one occasion: *'Mum asked me* (Trevor) *to go with her to visit Sheila – I was about 17 at the time. I said I would go and if she* (Sheila) *recognised me I would go again – but she had no recognition of me and just scarpered off after only a few minutes – I remember seeing her for the last time. I often thought about her and that I should have gone again. They were difficult times for all of us; I was engaged to be married and I was scared we might have children like Sheila'.*

Trevor and his fiancée, Marilyn sought help from their family doctor about their worries and both had tests to investigate if they were likely to carry the gene for PKU. This was long before the molecular genetics had been worked out and the test which was undertaken at BCH was a phenylalanine loading test. In this test a high dose of pure phenylalanine was given by mouth and blood levels measured over the next few hours to see if there was any evidence of reduced metabolism which might suggest carrier status. They remember the test and going to the hospital laboratory about five times in one day for blood tests each time. The results suggested that Trevor was unlikely to be a carrier but that Marilyn was more at risk of carrier status. Happily they have a son and daughter who do not have PKU.

The two younger brothers, Philip and Liam felt they never really got to know Sheila as she was already living at Chelmsley when they were growing up. Philip was away in children's homes with his two elder brothers in his early years and had not really understood what had happened to Sheila when she went to Chelmsley. The three brothers were away at the time when Sheila was admitted and when they got back she had just gone with no explanation. Mary was trying to protect her sons.

Looking at the photographs of Sheila when she was on the diet they remark: *'she looks lovely – bright and alert – she looks normal'.* They fondly recall the picture their Mum had of Sheila at home on the wall, at their home in Aston, in her green jumper and smiling. It is the photograph on the cover of this book and it was there all the time in their home as a reminder of their sister – never forgotten. When Trevor looked at the later picture when Sheila was in Chelmsley, nearly 40 years of age (p.81) – *'I couldn't "see" my sister as I used too – she was a complete stranger'.*

It was only years later after Sheila had died that her brothers began to understand something about what had happened at the Children's Hospital all those years ago. They had never had things explained and had not seen the film which Dr Bickel had made and even now find it very emotional and difficult to watch their sister during the treatment trial when she was only two years of age. In some ways there is disbelief about what happened to their family and the interest which others now have in their story. There is also an appreciation of what their Mum went through to do her best for Sheila during all those years as they were growing up and getting on with their own lives as best they could. '*I never helped our Mum as much as I should have*' is an understandable feeling. '*It must have been hard for our Mum, we should have helped more*'.

What about now? Sheila's brothers feel proud of what their Mother and Sheila contributed for the benefit of others, but it doesn't change what happened to Sheila and the effects it had on Mary and the rest of their family. The contrast with what can be provided for families with PKU today in 2019 is stark. There will be many other stories, with similar feelings from other families, and what could be said by Sheila's brothers could be said for all those untreated or late treated persons with PKU around the world. The brothers' own words best sum up their family story:

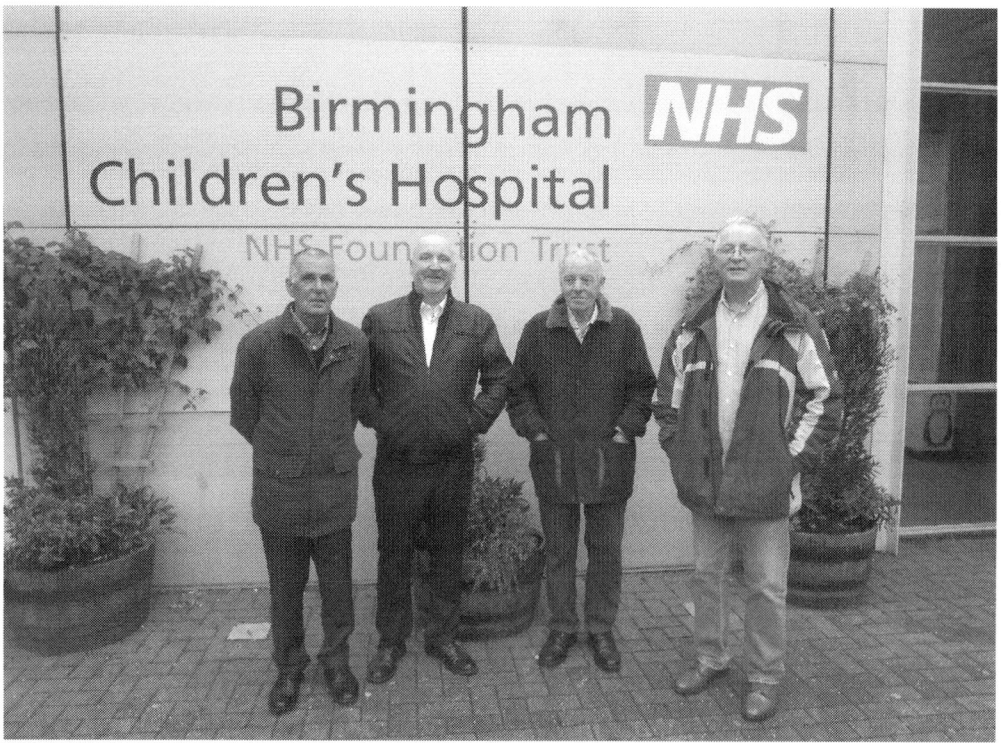

Sheila's Brothers at BCH, December 2016.

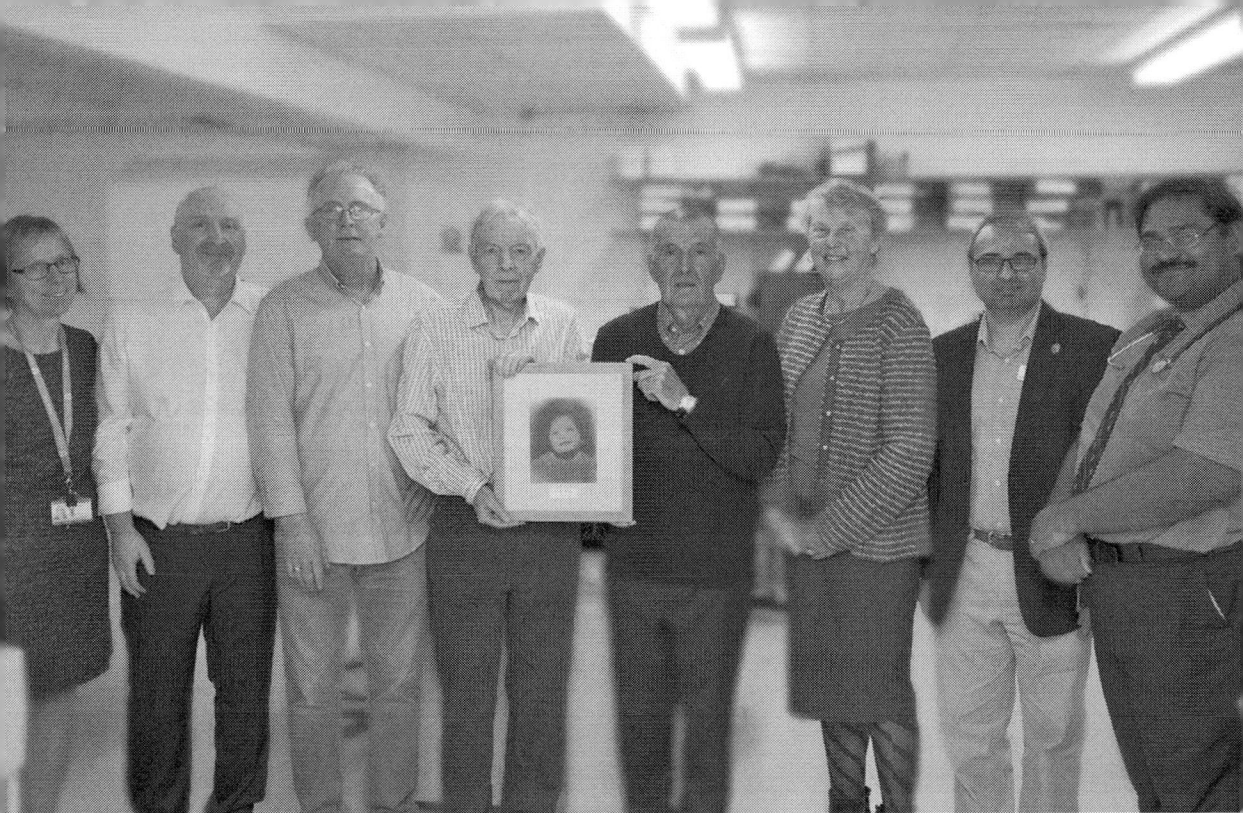

Sheila's Brothers with Author and Members of BCH Staff in the Newborn Screening Laboratory, December 2016. From left to right: Mary Anne Preece (Director of Newborn Screening), Liam, Philip, Trevor, Terry, Dr Anne Green, Dr Satish Rao (Deputy Medical Director), Dr Saikat Santra (Consultant in IMD).

- It was a fight a real struggle to give Sheila the diet
- Sheila loved tea – by the gallon – a lasting memory
- It used to scare me visiting Sheila
- It broke Mum; she must have had it hard
- Mum had a lot of part time jobs and lodgers
- I was scared of having children like Sheila
- Sheila was special because she was the only girl
- It would have been nice to have a sister who was normal
- We had nothing but we were happy
- Mum kept us together

In December 2016 Terry, Trevor, Philip and Liam visited the new Children's Hospital at Steelhouse Lane in Birmingham to see the glass column, full of charcoal, which had been used to prepare the diet for Sheila and see the commemorative items displayed in the laboratory. A framed photograph of Sheila was added to the collection.

14

CONCLUDING COMMENTS

Trevor Jones: *'Sheila and Mum showed that it could be done'*.

The history of any speciality is hallmarked by pioneers and for PKU there are none more important as those who contributed to this story. The impact from this work undertaken in the early 1950s has had huge benefits for individuals and families with PKU across the world and the low phenylalanine diet remains the standard treatment for PKU. The successful treatment we have today, so that those with PKU can lead normal lives, started with this story from Birmingham Children's Hospital with the pioneering work to prepare a diet for the first time.

It illustrates the importance of professionals working not as individuals but together as a team for the benefit of patients and families. There are many factors which contributed to and enabled all this to happen and in particular Leonard Parsons' role was pivotal in the careers of all three pioneers at BCH. He had the foresight to see the need for a hospital laboratory providing chemical investigations for children, which was brought to fruition with the appointment of Evelyn Hickmans. He encouraged John Gerrard to take up Paediatrics and attracted Horst Bickel to come and work in Birmingham because of his interest in amino acids. We should remember and give credit to Louis Woolf, working at Great Ormond Street Hospital, for his generosity as a true scientist in his willingness to share his ideas and to help the Birmingham team in their endeavours; this was without doubt a critical contribution.

The story also emphasizes the importance of doctors listening to a parent in their role of bringing about important developments. Without Mary Jones' perseverance and courage this might never have happened. Mary's determination is one which other parents will have felt and continue to feel – there MUST be some help from somewhere. There are many emotions which sum up what Mary must have gone through for all those years as she did her best for Sheila. Her courage to try a completely unproven diet for her daughter, extremely unpleasant and not without risk, and her determination and strength to continue to give it to Sheila for five years says so much about her. Mary's decision to seek care for Sheila at the age of nine years must have brought some relief knowing that her

14. Concluding Comments

daughter was going to be cared for, but also guilt and anger because she was having to leave her. In the book 'The Child who never grew' (Pearl Buck 1951) similar feelings are described by another mother who movingly and eloquently wrote about her own suffering and experiences with her mentally deficient daughter who eventually was diagnosed with PKU; in this book the author *'asks parents not to despair or turn away in shame'*. If Mary could have read these words they would have had real meaning and been of some comfort as she adjusted to the situation of leaving Sheila at Chelmsley.

During the treatment there was an enormous family sacrifice over many years as Sheila's needs dominated the family life. The whole family endured hardship with the social background at the time having a huge impact on their lives. Mary herself undoubtedly suffered with her mental health but it was for the love of her daughter and her family which enabled her to maintain Sheila's care for so long at home and to keep the family together. Sheila's brothers also had a hard and difficult life whilst their mother had to spend so much time looking after Sheila. The requirements of the dietary treatment were a huge load on them all. At nine years of age Sheila went into care at Chelmsley – for Mary this would be associated with some relief which allowed her to recover from the unrelenting stress and spend more time with her sons, but also sadness and maybe guilt. For her brothers they had lost a sister. Terry and Trevor were now 14 and 11 years of age and had grown up with Sheila and she was suddenly not there.

This is a story which deservedly belongs to Sheila as we acknowledge the enormous contribution which she unknowingly made. Taking an extremely unpleasant mixture as her main source of protein for the best part of five years, extensive periods of hospitalisation, separation from her mother and brothers for long periods, numerous blood and urine collections plus other consequences we can at best only begin to imagine. We don't really know why Sheila stopped taking the diet at the age of six to seven years but it seems likely it was quite simply too difficult to continue with it for any longer. In the early 1960s the current thinking was that it would be impractical to keep a young child with PKU on the diet at school age. It was only in the 1970s that studies confirmed early stopping was associated with cognitive decline, and later an association with more subtle defects. Although with our current knowledge diet for life is accepted – this was not so in 1955. Sheila struggled when being given the mixture and this would have got more difficult as she got older and stronger. The improvements in her developments had not been so great and her behaviour had become increasingly problematic. It was not clear that she would get any better and we now know that the treatment was started too late to make a real difference. Maybe Mary had begun to feel that it was all too late as she had to cope with Sheila's difficulties day in day out with no respite.

Mary had her four sons to consider and quite simply couldn't continue with no one around to help. She did what was best for Sheila and her family. We should also remember the practicalities of obtaining the diet in those early days. It was not possible for the hospital laboratory to continue to make the diet long term, and although commercial products were becoming available there would have been a cost implication not just to the NHS but also to families. Mary would not be able to afford to buy special foods or the costs of travel for the hospital visits. All these factors contributed to why Sheila did not continue with the treatment.

For those in the UK and with experience of working in the NHS it is hard to consider that Sheila was born only one year after the establishment of the NHS and her pioneering treatment took place only three years later. It was deservedly remembered as part of the 70th anniversary celebrations of the NHS

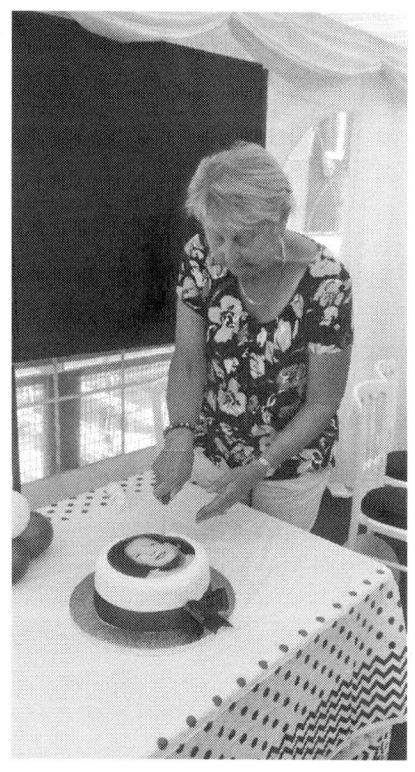

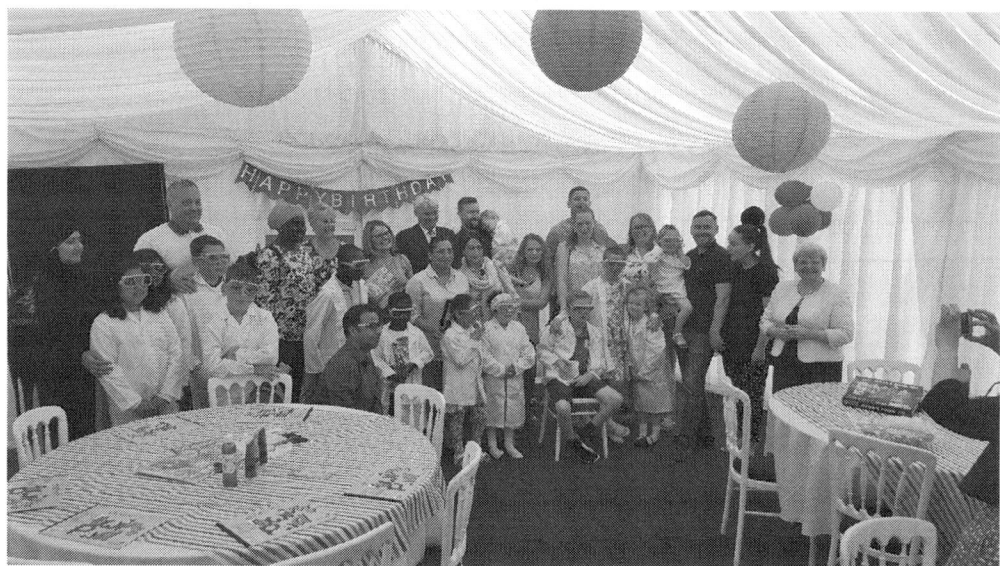

A Celebration of 70 years of the NHS and of Sheila's legacy at BCH in July 2018.

14. Concluding Comments

which took place at BCH in July 2018. Several of us, including those with PKU and other metabolic disorders and their families, participated. As the children enjoyed the party we remembered Sheila and tried to imagine what it would be like if PKU could not be treated so successfully today and what life would be like for so many families. 2019 marks the 50th anniversary of the introduction of PKU screening in the UK. The advances in our understanding and practices over the years has been huge.

As this story draws to an end and we look at the photograph of Sheila on the cover of this book – a pretty smiling little girl and look at the film made when she was four years old sat on her Mum's knee, building a tower with bricks and scribbling with a crayon, we cannot help but wonder what might have been if she had benefited from newborn screening and modern day treatment for PKU. How different life might have been for the Jones family; a sister for her brothers to play with and grow up with, and for Mary none of those nine years with all the stress and toil looking after a child with such severe disabilities on her own at home. Sheila was never able to realise her potential unlike those who have had life changing interventions not just for PKU but for many other disorders both genetic and non-genetic. The diet was started too late for Sheila, and the family circumstances and the social backdrop of the post war era were all against it making a difference for her. There will be many individuals with PKU like Sheila where treatment was never started, or diet discontinued early in the belief that the risk of further damage was over, or with poor control of the diet. These families will also share the same mixed emotions about their circumstances and what might have been.

This is a story of scientific innovation and of pioneering doctors who had the courage to try a completely unproven diet in a two year old child. It is also a story of a mother with determination, perseverance and love for her family. It is a story of family hardship and sadness that Sheila herself couldn't benefit from the diet. Importantly it is a story of a family who have such pride about what Mary and Sheila achieved and their legacy which now benefits so many. Telling Sheila's story doesn't change what happened in her life, but can bring a greater understanding for the family and a greater appreciation to those who now benefit from her legacy as she unlocked the treatment for PKU.

AFTERWORD

It is sometimes thought that clinical practice and public health are on different planets but this wonderful book clearly demonstrates how they are two sides of the one coin. A hypothesis was generated by looking at one child, then at a number of children with learning difficulties, the hypothesis was tested at laboratories and a treatment method was developed. With an understanding of the metabolism it was also possible to diagnose the disease accurately and this of course led to the development of a National Screening Programme for Phenylketonuria.

Birmingham can be proud of the part it has played in the history of global health by understanding and then taking action to tackle this dreadful condition. Clinical practice and public health are like threads running in different directions but combining to make the tapestry of healthcare.

Professor Sir Muir Gray, University of Oxford
Former Director of the UK National Screening Committee

January 2020

APPENDICES

Appendix I:

History of Birmingham

Birmingham is currently the second largest city in the UK and is located in the centre of England with a population of almost 1.1 million (Birmingham City Council 2011). In 2019 it is a vibrant city with a diverse multicultural population influenced by immigration from all over the world, most recently the Indian subcontinent and African America, a far cry from its small beginnings.

It originated in the 12th century as a small Saxon village with a market which attracted merchants and craftsmen particularly for the wool and leather industries. The population grew dramatically during the 16th and 17th centuries and it became a busy little town with a population of around 5,000 by 1650. The growth, initially from the merchant trade, was continued with the arrival of the manufacturing industry in the latter part of the 17th century, and by the 18th century Birmingham had become the leading metal manufacturer in the UK with approximately 30,000 inhabitants. Industry continued to boom together with its wealth and employment opportunities, and by 1801 (first census) Birmingham had a population of about 73,000 and became connected to other parts of the country with the building of canals and railways. It is said there are more canals than in Venice! Throughout the 19th century industry was still dominated by metalworking but other industries also emerged and the town became famous for jewellery, glass making and of course Cadbury's chocolate! Birmingham also became an important car manufacturing city in the late 19th and early 20th century and in 1905 The Austin Car Motor Company was born, located in Longbridge, south west of the city centre. Around this time the boundaries were extended to incorporate other surrounding villages and by 1930 the city had a population of around 1 million that remained at this level throughout the 1950s (Census, 1951). Throughout the 20th century, the immigrants from Ireland were Britain's largest foreign-born population.

With the outbreak of the Second World War *'The Austin'* car factory soon had to diversify production. The same machines and staff that had previously manufactured cars took in their stride the production of a whole range of intricate items/parts for the nation's war machine. The variety and quantities of articles produced were staggering, from steel helmets to aircraft and everything in between. As a major manufacturing centre the city had been an obvious target for enemy action with large parts destroyed by bombing and more than 2000 people being killed. As a result of this devastation inner city housing provision was poor and many families lived in poverty. There was a severe shortage of housing and a survey in 1954 showed that over 20% of homes were unfit for human habitation. A particular feature of Birmingham, like other Victorian cities, were the back-to-back houses (Chinn 2013, Rudge and Joseph 2015). Many thousands of these dwellings were built from the late 18th century for the rapidly increasing population as Birmingham grew from a large market town to a city. They were built as cheap housing for the working classes. There was poor sanitation, with toilets and water supplies shared between multiple households in enclosed courtyards (officially known as courts). Back-to-backs gained a poor reputation for inadequate levels of health and hygiene and around the mid-19th century this form of housing was deemed unsatisfactory and a hazard to health.

The passage of the Public Health Act 1875 permitted Corporations to ban building of new back-to-backs. However by the beginning of the 20th century, although no more of this type of housing was being built, there were still around 40,000 of such houses in Birmingham, accommodating about 200,000 people. After WWII most back-to-backs in the large cities were demolished as part of the slum clearances but in Birmingham it was not until the very end of the 1960s that the final families moved out. In Birmingham a single example has been retained and is administered by the National Trust as an historic museum.

In the early 1950s few people had cars and public transport within the city comprised Corporation buses and trams, although trams were discontinued in 1953. Some post war food rationing continued until 1954. These were difficult times.

Appendix II:

History of Birmingham Hospitals

As the town's population increased in the 17th and 18th centuries there was a growing need for somewhere to treat and look after the sick. The first hospitals in Birmingham, like those of most large cities in the UK, were created by a combination of voluntary and official initiatives. These early hospitals as we know them today, i.e. as a place for the sick to be cared for, were part of the city's workhouse provision (Poor Law Act of 1601) with the first workhouse in Birmingham opening in 1733. The workhouse was essentially where the poor and the homeless were housed but also catered for the sick. The workhouses could not meet the growing needs from overcrowded houses with increasing sickness and in 1766 the 'Infirmary' wing was added to the Birmingham workhouse. In 1779 the first dedicated hospital, the General Hospital, opened in the city centre with just forty beds. In parallel with the workhouse provision for the sick, medical education was beginning with the first clinical teaching for medical apprentices taking place at the new General Hospital.

Under the subsequent Poor Law Act of 1834 every parish had to provide workhouses for its destitute and sick population but some parishes had insufficient means to make provision, and so they united with neighbours to form Unions for this purpose. These workhouses and the hospitals continued to be under huge pressure as Birmingham's population grew further. In 1851 a new infirmary building was constructed and opened on the Dudley Road workhouse site as the Birmingham Union Workhouse and Infirmary. This subsequently became Dudley Road Hospital and currently exists as the City Hospital. Other new hospitals were established during the 19th century with the opening of the Queen's Hospital in 1841 as a teaching hospital and several specialist institutions including those for disorders of the Ear, Nose and Throat (1877); Eye (1824); Orthopaedic (1817) and Women (1871).

A specialist Children's Hospital in Birmingham opened in 1862 and was one of only a few specialist children's hospitals established in the UK in the 1800s. Great Ormond Street Hospital, London was the first to be opened in 1851 with others in Liverpool, Manchester and Edinburgh following. The Birmingham and Midland Free Hospital for Sick Children was opened in the city centre on Steelhouse Lane. It was initially opened only as an outpatient department with the inpatient department of just 16 beds following a fortnight later! It soon expanded to 33 beds but services needed to grow further and in 1869 a new site in Broad Street was acquired that allowed the construction of an isolation block which opened in 1877. This was badly needed to cope with the increasing numbers of children with infectious diseases at that time. In 1907 the premises and the building were now deemed not fit for purpose for the sick children of the city and the governors resolved to build a new hospital, with the foundation stone for the new hospital at the Ladywood site being laid on St George's Day, 23rd April 1913. The hospital was formally opened on 21st May 1919 by King George V and Queen Mary.

The Queen Elizabeth Hospital opened in 1938 with commencement of teaching of medical students, this being the foundation of the Birmingham Medical School. There was then a period of further expansion of the hospitals and closure of the old workhouses. Medical progress had made so many demands in terms of staff, equipment and services that it was becoming impossible to run the hospitals on a purely voluntary basis and this arrangement could not have continued without intervention from the state. The voluntary hospitals were under pressure of financial stringency and were becoming aware of the advantages of a planned coordinated hospital service and so it was in 1948 that the National Health Service (NHS) was created.

Appendix III:

Learning Disability Services in the UK

The provision of services and care for those individuals with learning disabilities who have mental health and behaviour problems has gone through huge changes. There has also been a succession of changing terminology which has happened in parallel with changes in the organisation of services.

The Lunacy Act and Asylums

Mental Health services in the UK before the establishment of the NHS in 1948 were governed by the 1890 Lunacy Act. The Lunacy Act formed the basis of mental health law in England and Wales from 1890 until 1959. It placed an obligation on local authorities to maintain institutions for the mentally ill. It made no distinction between individuals with mental illness and those with learning disability and all individuals were referred to as 'lunatics'. Large institutions or 'asylums' were established across the country. The Lunacy Act set the parameters for admission and a legal framework whereby an individual had to be declared 'insane' in order to be admitted to the asylum. Under this Act asylums became a last resort for those with mental illness rather than a means for treatment/recovery. There was no legislative procedure for patients who wished to be treated voluntarily at that time.

Most asylums were built on the outskirts of major cities, isolated from local communities – Birmingham was no exception. They provided a 'rural retreat' for patients and most operated as self-sufficient communities with their own water supply, farm, laundry etc. They were deliberately located away from the rest of the community rather than within the city.

Classification of Individuals with Mental Deficiency

In the early 1900s the language changed and the terms 'mental deficiency' and 'mental defective' were formally established by the 1913 Mental Deficiency Act. A Board of Control for Lunacy and Mental Deficiency to oversee the implementation of services was established. Individuals were classified into one of four categories based on their degree and type of mental impairment.

Idiots – *those with the most severe mental defectiveness, unable to guard against common physical dangers.*

Imbeciles – *those with mental defectiveness not amounting to idiocy but who are unable to take care of themselves or, in the case of children being unable to be taught to do so.*

Feeble Minded persons – *those with mental defectiveness not amounting to imbecility but requiring care, supervision and control for protection of themselves or others, and, in the case of children being unable to benefit from instruction in ordinary schools.*

Moral Imbeciles – *where mental defectiveness is coupled with vicious and criminal tendencies thus requiring care, supervision and control for the protection of others.*

The diagnosis for individuals into one of these categories was often arrived at after a period of institutionalised care or via the law courts. Responsibility for care of individuals in these categories rested with the local authority and there was a special person employed to oversee the process of medical assessment and certification before presenting to the magistrate for consideration for admission. Once accepted, arrangements would be made for the individual to be taken to the local institution.

During the early 1900s there was a rising number of individuals in society with poorly understood and untreatable conditions resulting in mental deficiency. These included lead poisoning, syphilis, tumours, congenital malformations and an emerging group of patients with metabolic disorders – including those with Phenylketonuria (PKU). These individuals, although rare, added to the growing numbers who presented for admission to asylums, albeit the cause of their condition was usually unknown. 40% of the PKU cases would have been considered imbeciles (moderate learning disability) and the rest as idiots (severe learning disability). These terms continued to be used until the 1970s.

We could not conceive today of using such names. Idiots, imbeciles, and feeble-minded people would be retrospectively regarded as having severe, moderate and mild learning deficiencies.

Development of Psychiatric Services

There was initially no legislative procedure for patients to be admitted voluntarily to an asylum although some individual institutions had made their own arrangements. This *ad hoc* voluntary admission procedure was extended to other institutions in 1930 resulting in an ever-increasing asylum population. This simultaneously encouraged establishment of outpatient services and was the beginning of community-based psychiatric services.

By 1938 approximately 150 000 individuals were institutionalised in local authority mental hospitals across England, Wales and Scotland. In 1948 these services became part of the newly created National Health Service (NHS) and by 1953 nearly half the NHS beds were for mental defects or those with mental illness.

The Mental Health Act 1959

The Mental Deficiency Act of 1913 remained in place until it was replaced by the Mental Health Act 1959. This provided a new legal framework for the treatment and care of people with learning disabilities. The major changes were clarification of why an individual might need to be admitted and treated against their will and the distinction between voluntary and involuntary treatments became clearer. The Act stated that patients should only be admitted on an involuntary basis unless they were a danger to themselves or others, a procedure subsequently known as being '*sectioned*'. New terminology introduced by the Mental Health Act to describe individuals were 'subnormal' and 'severely subnormal', replacing the previously used mental defective and mental deficiency (using a definition of 'arrested' or 'incomplete' development of the mind).

Education was still not a right and only with the 1970 Education Act did education became universal for those with mental deficiency. Until then such individuals were described as 'ineducable', a term introduced by the earlier 1944 Education Act.

Whilst the new Mental Health Act emphasised the importance of enabling 'mentally ill' people to live, as far as possible, in the community it did not make the provision of appropriate facilities. Consequently, large numbers of individuals continued to be housed in the former asylums and workhouses which then became large psychiatric hospitals. Nationally, at this time, psychiatric hospitals housed 40% of total NHS patients but received only 20% of the NHS budget and were deemed a 'Cinderella' service. The generally poor standards of care and quality of life in these hospitals fuelled a political and social movement in the early 1960s to close down these large Victorian institutions and deinstitutionalise the thousands of individuals within them by caring for them in the community.

As a result of the 'Care in the Community' Consultative Document Study in 1981, the policy of community care became accepted with changes to enable care in an individual's own home or in small community-based establishments. It however took a long time to fully implement this policy and many of these large hospitals did not close until well into the 1990s.

Birmingham's Psychiatric Hospitals

In line with the national picture, there were several large Victorian institutions in Birmingham for those with mental deficiency. Most had started life as workhouses in the late 1800s and by the 1960s had become large psychiatric hospitals housing over 5000 patients in overcrowded, dilapidated conditions. Two of these institutions in Birmingham are relevant to this story: **Chelmsley Hospital, Marston Green** and **Highcroft Hospital, Erdington** (see Map Birmingham, 9 and 10).

All of these psychiatric hospitals in Birmingham eventually closed and have since been demolished or developed for housing/businesses with patients being rehoused in smaller community-based units or cared for at home. For those with a learning disability requiring hospital treatment new psychiatric hospitals have been built, and in the case of Chelmsley a new hospital (Brooklands) was built on part of the original Chelmsley Hospital site.

The language for mental health continued to evolve and by the time of the Mental Health Act 1983 the term 'subnormality' was replaced by 'mental impairment'. The term 'mental handicap' (mild, moderate and severe) was widely used until the 1990s when the Department of Health promoted the term 'people with learning disabilities'.

Appendix IV:

Extracts from Personal Notes

These unidentified notes (some handwritten, others typed) are part of the historical records of the Clinical Chemistry Department, BCH. They all concern PKU and are assumed to have been written by various professionals. The originals form part of the BCH Archive. A descriptive summary of the content of each set is provided below together with selected extracts in *italics*.

Set 1: The Story of Phenylketonuria
Handwritten notes probably by Evelyn Hickmans – c.1960s.

Includes history and chemical basis of PKU with description of clinical features of 12 PKU patients and history of Sheila and her diet. Refers to availability of commercial dietary products and newborn screening in Birmingham and across Great Britain (GB) using Phenistix.

Description of 12 patients
At birth, children appear to be normal, but in a short time show signs of (being) *mental backwards*
Hair – fair and course – rather like tow
A musty – mouse like smell
Have jerky, unco-ordinated movements, therefore cannot pick up toys – or walk or may be stand. Very backward
Skin – coarse-dry-eczema
If condition is not corrected they have IQ's ?<10, Adults have mental age of about 3 years
Usually well-built and physically strong and live to adult life
But unable to feed themselves and keep themselves clean etc. They cannot be 'house-trained'. Incontinent

Urine test with Ferric Chloride
Back in 1951, we at the CHB (Children's Hospital Birmingham) were regularly detecting amino acids by chromatography. So that when the RMO found a child in his clinic, whom he thought after a preliminary test of the urine with Ferric Chloride, was a PKU case, we were quickly able to confirm the presence of excess phenylalanine in the urine. The child was admitted and began an investigation and lasted for a period of 2 years 1951-1953.

Sheila
This little patient, Sheila about 2 years old was admitted October 1951 and found to have all the described symptoms.

She could not stand, walk nor talk

Showed no interest in food or surroundings

Lay in cot, moaning and crying, banging head on pillow and rolling from side to side till hair was nearly worn off at the back and sides

Fair hair like tow

Rough skin and eczema

Characteristic smell

Exaggerated movements

The child was sent home on this carefully calculated diet sheet – the mother carrying (hugging) a Winchester full of the 'medicine' as well as this rather heavy and awkward little girl. She returned each week for ferric chloride tests and chromatograms and occasional plasma content of phenylalanine.

Finally it was decided that perhaps Sheila was too old to benefit from this dietary treatment to any extent and that the treatment should be started on patients as soon as possible after birth if only they could be found.

Where treatment began in the early weeks of life, success has been registered in 80% cases. It was thought that these patients might have to partake of a low phenylalanine diet all their lives but some have been put on to a normal diet after 5-6-7 years and the results have shown no mental deterioration.

Phenistix screening
Estimated incidence 1 per 20,000, 40 cases per year in GB where cases have been proved (and this is done carefully in hospital). They are supplied with a low phenylalanine preparation in solid form. The trouble is that this 'flour' is difficult to cook and very nasty to taste.

Set 2: PKU and Dietary treatment
Handwritten notes probably by Evelyn Hickmans – 1964.

These include general notes on PKU in particular detailing the chemistry and chemical structures of phenylalanine metabolism. The notes contain chemical formulae and abbreviations with calculations which would suggest the author is a chemist. The metabolic pathway for phenylalanine is drawn out for the blackboard. It is likely they were notes for a lecture – as Cheltenham 1964 is mentioned. There are references to 'our' and 'we' in relation to Sheila, and as well as familiarity with chemistry and an understanding of nutrition which strongly suggests they were written by Evelyn Hickmans.

Appendix IV

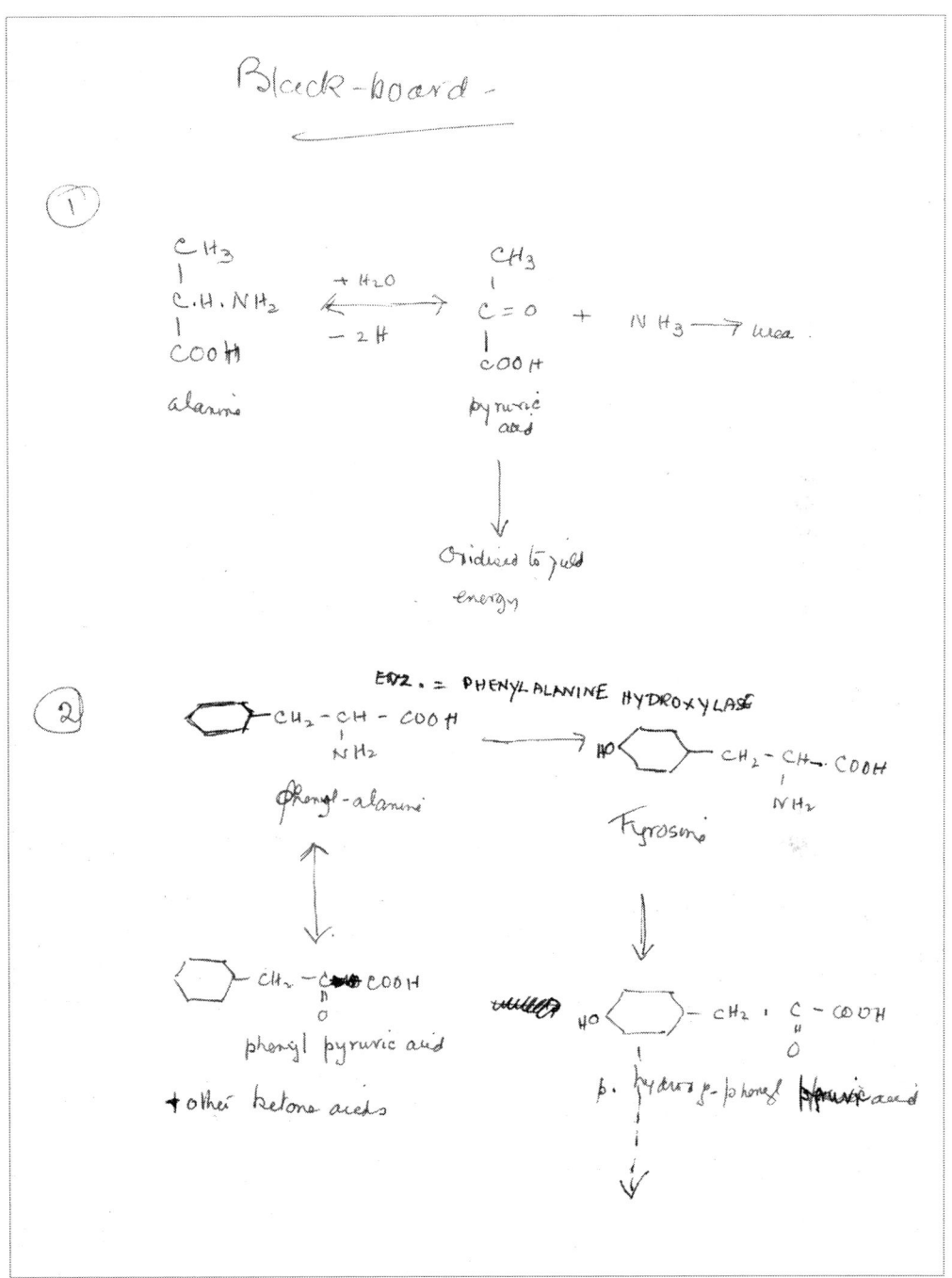

Set 2: Original lecture notes.

Sheila

Sheila's presentation – details similar to those in set 1.

In October 1951 we were familiar with chromatographic method of detecting AA (amino acids). So were very pleased when the RMO (Resident Medical Officer) came to us and said he had a mentally backward child whose urine gave olive-green colour with ferric chloride and that it might be a PKU. Ferric chloride gives a distinct olive-green colour with phenylalanine. The patient was admitted. All the routine tests were normal but 2 way paper chromatograms confirmed the presence of excessive amounts of phenylalanine in the urine, but of no other amino acids. The blood level was also raised.

Preparation of phenylalanine free food

There is detail about the production of the phenylalanine free food. Specific reference is made of the cost of adding the l- amino acids to the charcoal treated casein hydrolysate. There is discussion of the newborn screening started in Birmingham in 1959 and the treatment of younger infants. There is information on phenylalanine requirements and dietary calculations.

Since these children (PKUics) cannot metabolise phenylalanine it was decided to try to supply a diet with a low content of phenylalanine in it sufficient to keep the blood level normal, if it could be prepared. As all protein contains phenylalanine, protein as such could not be given except in limited amounts. Since casein contains all AA which go to make up complex proteins we started with acid casein hydrolysate and decided to try to remove the phenylalanine – thus leaving a residue equivalent to milk protein without phenylalanine. A 10% solution of acid casein hydrolysate was treated with acidified charcoal first by stirring in beakers, then by pouring it through columns of charcoal, till the filtrate was free of phenylalanine. Each batch was tested by chromatography and as chromatograms showed that some tyrosine, tryptophan and cysteine had also been removed these were added as pure amino acids – <u>very expensive.</u> Final volume was made up so that 100ml = 10g protein. The diet is distasteful and monotonous. After 6 months on this diet the patient became brighter, less fractious and awkward, and took more interest in her food and surroundings. She could crawl, stand with the help of a chair. Hair improved, skin improves and she lost her mouse like smell. She gained weight but mental condition was not obviously improved. Further mention is made of Sheila and that *the patient was no better* and *that possibly treatment had begun too late. Sheila's mother had succumbed to all her worries looking after her children for so long and is now in a mental hospital suffering from a complete mental breakdown. Sheila is also in retreat.*

A few commercial firms were persuaded to make the necessary phenylalanine free preparations and a number of such preparations in powder form are now available to PKU patients.

Appendix IV

Since 1953 reports from Birmingham and other centres show that mental improvement depends on early recognition since few children not treated before 3 yr of age show improvement in mental condition.

Set 3: The story of Phenylketonuria – an inborn error of metabolism
Handwritten notes (two versions) c.1962 – Unidentified? Dr Gerrard.

The notes include a quote from Professor Squire 1962, University of Birmingham:

'Ultimately perhaps when the true nature of many more specific defects underlying mental disorders becomes sufficiently understood this will turn out to be the most important result (our attitude of benefitting a proportion of mentally handicapped children) of these researchers conducted 10 years ago at Birmingham Children's Hospital'.

Set 4: No Title by Dr Horst Bickel
Typed notes subsequently published as part of publication: Bickel H Phenylketonuria: Past, Present and Future J in Metab Dis 3, 1980, pp.123-132.

Sheila our patient was badly brain damaged, could not sit nor stand and took no interest in her food or her surroundings. She had fair hair, eczema and a typical mouse-like smell. The mother was of course in despair and could not share our excitement about the rare diagnosis, nor our interest in the strong phenylalanine spot on the chromatogram. Instead she waited for me every morning before the laboratory door, making quite clear that treatment was what she wanted for her child not fancy investigations. She did not accept that so far there was no therapy for this condition.

The mother's perseverance gave me no chance to rest on the strength of a fine diagnosis, so I started to wonder if there might not be a causal relation between the phenylalanine excess and the child's brain damage and – in a primitive way of thinking – whether one could not improve her condition by getting rid of the phenylalanine spot on the chromatogram by limiting the phenylalanine intake in the food.

Set 5: Interview with Dr Hickmans
Typed notes of Dr N. Raine and Dr R. Gaddie interview with Dr Hickmans about her career at BCH c.1960s.

'I had two assistants to help with the chromatography. Three of us worked day and night on chromatography otherwise we would never have got the work done'.

Appendix V:

The John Scott Award
Documents and Letters

This appendix lists documents relating to this event which are included in the BCH Archive; selected ones are reproduced as part of the appendix.

John Scott Award 1962
1. Notification of the Award
a) City of Philadelphia, 1962. *Letter to Professor Gerrard notification of the Award* [letter] (Personal communication 19 June 1962) Birmingham: BCH Archive.

2. Letters of Congratulations
a) Squire, J., 1962. *Letter of Congratulations to Dr Hickmans.* [letter] (Personal communication, 5 July 1962). Birmingham: BCH Archive.
b) Hubble, D., 1962. *Letter of Congratulations to Dr Hickmans.* [letter] (Personal communication, 9 July 1962). Birmingham: BCH Archive.
c) Norton, E.A., 1962. *Letter of Congratulations to Dr Hickmans.* [letter] (Personal communication, 16 July 1962). Birmingham: BCH Archive.

3. Letters concerning Scientific Meeting and Award ceremony
a) Association of Clinical Biochemists, 1962. Wilkinson, J.H. 1962. *Letter to Dr Hickmans about Scientific Meeting and Award Ceremony.* [letter] (Personal communication 2 July 1962). Birmingham: BCH Archive.
b) Association of Clinical Biochemists, 1962. Wilkinson, J.H. 1962. *Letter to Dr Hickmans concerning Scientific Meeting and Award Ceremony.* [letter] (Personal communication 9 July 1962). Birmingham: BCH Archive.
c) Association of Clinical Biochemists, 1962. Gaddie, R. *Letter concerning Scientific Meeting and Award Ceremony.* [letter] (Personal communication 12 July 1962). Birmingham: BCH Archive.
d) City of Philadelphia, 1962. *Letter to Dr Hickmans concerning Scientific Meeting and Award Ceremony.* [letter] (Personal communication 26 July 1962) Birmingham: BCH Archive.
e) City of Philadelphia, 1962. *Letter to Dr Hickmans concerning Scientific Meeting and Award Ceremony.* [letter] (Personal communication 22 August 1962) Birmingham: BCH Archive.

Appendix V

CITY OF PHILADELPHIA
BOARD OF DIRECTORS OF CITY TRUSTS

G. CURTIS PRITCHARD
SECRETARY

1601 SPRING GARDEN STREET
PHILADELPHIA 30, PENNA.
LOcust 8-7575

June 19, 1962

Professor John Gerrard
Department of Paediatrics
University of Saskatoon
Saskatchewan, Canada

Dear Sir:

    At a meeting of the

    BOARD OF DIRECTORS OF CITY TRUSTS

Friday, June 15, 1962, the following Resolution was adopted:

    RESOLVED-that, upon the recommendation of the Advisory Committee, the John Scott Award, with premiums indicated below, be made to the following:

Dr. Horst Bickle	$333.33
Professor John Gerrard	$333.33
Miss Evelyn Hickmans	$333.34

    For their invention of a method of controlling Phenyl ketonuria

    No definite plans for presenting the award to you have been formulated at this time. We have found it most appropriate to arrange for such a presentation before a scientific or professional society of which the recipient is a member. If you have any suggestions, they will be most welcome. I will keep you posted as to progress in this matter.

    Data which we will require from you includes (1) any degrees (up to two) which you would prefer to have engraved on the medal, and (2) a resume of your background which will be required in preparing the citation and the usual publicity releases.

    Looking forward to hearing from you and extending warmest congratulations,

Sincerely yours,

Curtis Pritchard
Secretary

rja

1a. Notification of the Award.

Sheila

TELEPHONE: SELLY OAK 0291
           "   " 1301

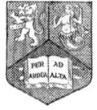

UNIVERSITY OF BIRMINGHAM

Prof. JOHN R. SQUIRE.

DEPARTMENT OF EXPERIMENTAL PATHOLOGY,
THE MEDICAL SCHOOL,
THE HOSPITALS CENTRE,
BIRMINGHAM, 15.

5th July, 1962.

Dear Dr. Hickmans,

    As I said over the telephone yesterday morning we are all absolutely delighted about the very great honour shown to you and your colleagues by the decision to make the John Scott Award to you for your work and discoveries. I saw Otto Wolff and Keith Rogers at lunch yesterday and they too were bubbling with pleasure and excitement.

    I have had a word with the Assistant Editor of the Birmingham Post as promised and he is to check with the University reporter, Mr. Clover, so as to ensure that no premature press release is made at this end. I was not too sure about the date when our American colleagues would be publishing the news but told him I hoped we should discover this in due course from you. I am sorry to have given you this additional bother. It does indeed seem appropriate that our local newspaper should carry the good news when it is eventually made public.

    Again our warmest congratulations and best wishes,

           Yours sincerely,

           John Squire

Dr. E. Hickmans,
The Corner House,
Castlecroft Gardens,
Finchfield,
Nr. Wolverhampton.

2a) Letters of Congratulations.

Appendix V

DVH/AMD

DEPARTMENT OF PAEDIATRICS AND CHILD HEALTH
Professor DOUGLAS HUBBLE, M.D., F.R.C.P.

O. H. WOLFF, M.A., M.D., M.R.C.P., D.C.H.
B. D. BOWER, M.D., M.R.C.P., D.C.H.
JUNE K. LLOYD, M.B., M.R.C.P., D.P.H.

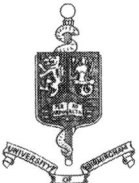

THE CHILDREN'S HOSPITAL,
LADYWOOD ROAD,
BIRMINGHAM 16.

TELEPHONE:
EDGBASTON 4851

9th July, 1962.

Miss E. Hickmans,
1, Castlecroft Gardens,
Wolverhampton.

Dear Miss Hickmans,

The news has just come through that you, together with Professor Bickel and Professor Gerrard have been given the John Scott Award by the City Trusts of Philadelphia, U.S.A. This is a great honour and the staff of the Children's Hospital here would wish to congratulate you upon it I am sure. Meanwhile I send these interim congratulations from the Professorial Unit. How delighted Sir Leonard Parsons and Professor Smellie would have been to have had this news.

With best wishes,

Yours sincerely,

Douglas Hubble

2b) Letters of Congratulations.

Sheila

THE UNITED BIRMINGHAM HOSPITALS

FROM
THE CHAIRMAN OF THE
BOARD OF GOVERNORS

THE QUEEN ELIZABETH HOSPITAL,
BIRMINGHAM, 15.

C

16th July 1962.

Dear Dr. Hickmans,

When the Board of Governors met on Friday last they were delighted to hear that the Board of Directors of the State Trustees of Philadelphia are resolved to confer upon you and your associates the John Scott award in recognition of your work on phenylketonuria at the Childrens' Hospital.

We recognise that there has as yet been no public announcement of this decision, but I was asked nevertheless to convey to you the warmest congratulations of the Board of Governors on this high distinction that you are to receive.

It is a special pleasure to us that this announcement is to be made in the centenary year of the history of the Childrens' Hospital, and I know that this public recognition of your invaluable services to the work of the hospital over so many years will give very great pleasure and satisfaction to your many friends in Birmingham.

With kind regards and good wishes,

Evan Ag. Norton.

Miss E. M. Hickmans, M.Sc., Ph.D.
The Corner House,
Castlecroft Gardens,
Wolverhampton.

2c) Letters of Congratulations.

Appendix V

THE ASSOCIATION OF CLINICAL BIOCHEMISTS

Hon. Secretary:
DR. J. H. WILKINSON,
WESTMINSTER MEDICAL SCHOOL,
HORSEFERRY ROAD,
LONDON, S.W.I.
Tel.: VICtoria 8161, Ext. 24.

Hon. Treasurer:
DR. R. GADDIE,
THE GENERAL HOSPITAL,
BIRMINGHAM, 4.
Tel.: Central 8611.

2nd July, 1962.

Miss E. M. Hickmans,
The Corner House,
Castlecroft Gardens,
Finchfield,
Nr. Wolverhampton.

Dear Miss Hickmans,

Many thanks for your letter of 28th June. I was delighted to hear that you have been awarded the John Scott Award for your work on Phenyl-ketonuria. Please accept my warmest congratulations.

I fully agree that if we could make arrangements for the presentation to be made at the meeting of the Association's Annual General Meeting in September, it would be most appropriate. I shall see if suitable arrangements can be made. You will appreciate that this is a joint meeting with the Association of Clinical Pathologists and the organisers will have to be consulted. I do not think there will be any difficulty and I shall write to you again as soon as I have heard from them.

I am sure that your colleagues in the A.C.B. will join me in congratulating you on this richly deserved honour.

Yours sincerely,

J. H. Wilkinson
Hon. Secretary.

P.S. I had a card from Dr. Gaddie recommending this procedure.

3a) Letters concerning Scientific Meeting and Award ceremony.

THE ASSOCIATION OF CLINICAL BIOCHEMISTS

Hon. Secretary:
DR. J. H. WILKINSON,
WESTMINSTER MEDICAL SCHOOL,
HORSEFERRY ROAD,
LONDON, S.W.I.
Tel.: VICtoria 8161, Ext. 24.

Hon. Treasurer:
DR. R. GADDIE,
THE GENERAL HOSPITAL,
BIRMINGHAM, 4.
Tel.: Central 8611.

9th July, 1962.

Miss E. M. Hickmans,
The Corner House,
Castlecroft Gardens,
Finchfield,
Nr. Wolverhampton.

Dear Miss Hickmans,

Thank you for your letter of July 6th. I think you are wise to suggest Birmingham as the most appropriate place for the presentation of the John Scott Award, and if you can make arrangements with your Regional Secretary I am sure that Council will be very happy to do anything to make the occasion successful. Please let me know if you would like me to take any further action.

Yours sincerely,

J. H. Wilkinson
Hon. Secretary.

3b) Letters concerning Scientific Meeting and Award ceremony.

Appendix V

THE ASSOCIATION OF CLINICAL BIOCHEMISTS

Hon. Secretary:
DR. J. H. WILKINSON,
WESTMINSTER MEDICAL SCHOOL,
HORSEFERRY ROAD,
LONDON, S.W.1.
Tel.: VICtoria 8161, Ext. 24.

Hon. Treasurer:
DR. R. GADDIE,
THE GENERAL HOSPITAL,
BIRMINGHAM, 4.
Tel.: Central 8611.

12th July, 1962

Dr. E. M. Hickmans,
   The Corner House,
      Castlecroft Gardens,
         Wolverhampton.

Dear Miss Hickmans,

        I got your letter this morning when I arrived back from holiday. It is disappointing that Wilkinson finds the programme for the London meeting already too full, and I shall raise the matter at the Council Meeting on Monday. Probably the reason is that the meeting is partly a joint one with the A.C.P. Anyhow, Birmingham is a more suitable place. The local secretary, Dr. Northam of this department and other members of the Midland Committee agree that it will be a great honour to have the meeting in Birmingham. He is writing to Philadelphia at once to see what arrangements they want made and we shall make the Bush lecture meeting fit their requirements. Whether the Children's Hospital has a large enough room I very much doubt but the details can be arranged after we hear from America.

      We had a very good holiday indeed, thank you.

      With kind regards,

         Yours sincerely,

         Robert Gaddie

3c) Letters concerning Scientific Meeting and Award ceremony.

Sheila

CITY OF PHILADELPHIA
BOARD OF DIRECTORS OF CITY TRUSTS

G. CURTIS PRITCHARD
SECRETARY

1601 SPRING GARDEN STREET
PHILADELPHIA 30, PENNA.
LOcust 8-7575

July 26, 1962

Evelyn M. Hickmans
The Corner House
Castlecroft Gardens
Finchfield, Nr. Wolverhampton
England

Dear Dr. Hickmans:

This will acknowledge, with thanks, receipt of yours dated July 16th.

It now appears that we will not be able to make all three presentations, to you, Dr. Bickel and Dr. Gerrard, at the same time.

We are writing to Dr. Northam to make arrangements to present your award to you around October 24th in Birmingham, as he suggested. I have written to Dr. Bickel and asked if he could be there to receive his award at the same time; however if he cannot make it, then we will arrange for his presentation at his convenience.

Dr. Gerrard will probably receive his award in Chicago around October 27th when he will be attending meetings of the American Academy of Pediatrics.

Thank you again for all your help and cooperation.

Sincerely yours,

G. Curtis Pritchard
Secretary

rja

3d) Letters concerning Scientific Meeting and Award ceremony.

Appendix V

CITY OF PHILADELPHIA
BOARD OF DIRECTORS OF CITY TRUSTS

G. CURTIS PRITCHARD
    SECRETARY

1601 SPRING GARDEN STREET
PHILADELPHIA 30, PENNA.
LOcust 8-7575

August 22, 1962

Evelyn M. Hickmans
The Corner House
Castlecroft Gardens
Finchfield, Nr. Wolverhampton
England

Dear Dr. Hickmans:

    We have now had word from Dr. Bickel that he would be very pleased to receive his John Scott Award in Birmingham on October 24th along with you.

    Dr. Gerrard has found that it will be impossible for him to come to England this fall, so we will arrange for his presentation at another time.

    Arrangements are now being made with Dr. Northam and the American Embassy in London to present the awards to you and Dr. Bickel on October 24th.

Sincerely yours,

Curtis Pritchard
Secretary

rja

3e) Letters concerning Scientific Meeting and Award ceremony.

4. Attendees at Scientific Meeting
a) Birmingham Children's Hospital, 1962. *John Scott Award Meeting and Ceremony October 24th 1962. List of Attendees.* [list] Birmingham: BCH Archive.

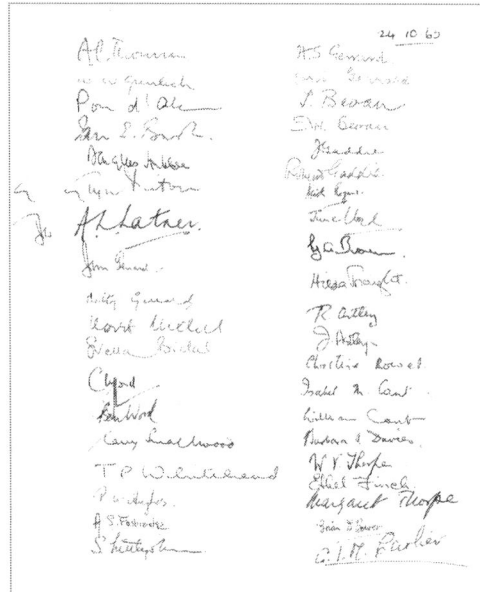
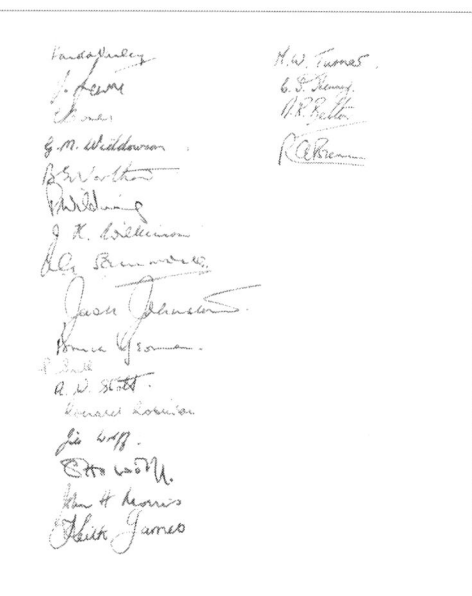
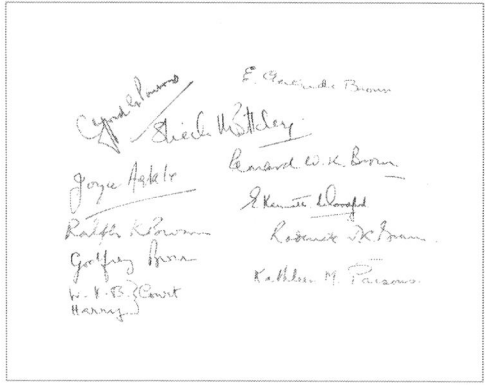

Signatures of Attendees.

Appendix V

5. Evening Celebrations at Staff House, University of Birmingham
a) *Dinner in Honour*, 1962. The Staff House, The University of Birmingham: BCH Archive.

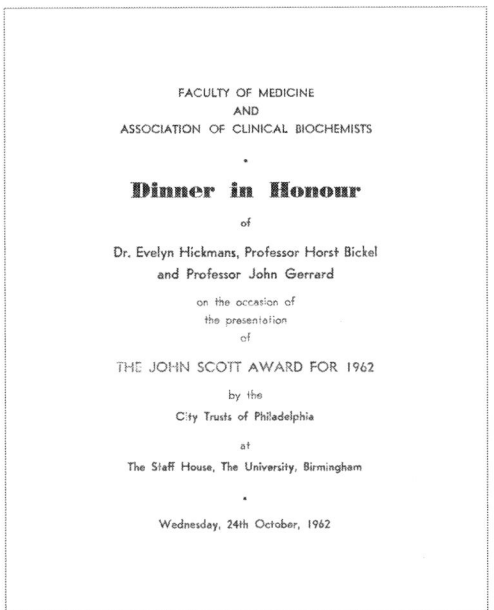
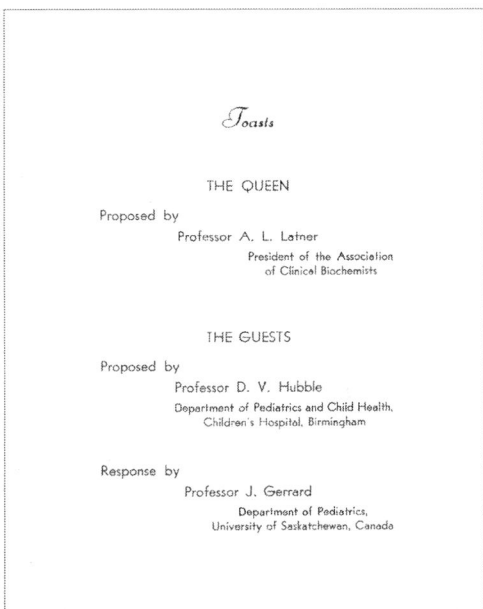

b) After Dinner Speech. Gerrard, J., 1962. *In Reply to Dr D.V. Hubble's Toast to the Guests.* [speech]). Birmingham: BCH Archive.

This speech was delivered at the evening dinner by Professor John Gerrard on behalf of himself, Professor Bickel and Dr Hickmans in reply to the toast by Professor D.V. Hubble to the guests. Those present included Professor A d'Abreu, Dean of the Faculty of Medicine and Sir Arthur Thompson, Vice Principal of Birmingham University. The speech is reproduced in full.

Ladies and Gentlemen, etc.

Dr Hickmans, Dr Bickel and I are all very grateful to you, not only for having brought us together again under such delightful circumstances, but also for the arrangements you made for the presentation of the award this afternoon, and for asking Professor Hubble to propose the toast to us, your guests, at this dinner so generously provided by the Medical Faculty and the Association of Clinical Biochemists, subsidised – I understand – in large measure by yourselves. The presence of so many of my old teachers, Sir Arthur Thompson for example, Dr Smallwood and Dr Parsons brings back many, many very happy memories and my presence here demonstrates, I hope that not all your teaching fell on stony ground.

Sheila

As you can well understand this occasion has brought great happiness and pleasure not only to the three of us, but also to our relatives – I am grateful to you for having made it possible for my mother and father, and also for an uncle and an aunt, who actually stood in loco parentis for many years, to be with us tonight, and Horst Bickel and I are more than delighted that our wives, Stella and Betty can be here too. But it is not only our relatives who have shared in our happiness for some of our old patients as well. Both Horst and I have heard for example, from our old friend Mrs Matthews whose son, David was admitted to the Children's Hospital in extremis when only three years old, with renal and bladder calculi due to cystinuria. Horst and Dr Baines rescued him from the jaws of death, and he is now a strapping lad of 15. We have not heard I am sorry to say, from Mrs Jones, the mother of the original Phenylketonuric, Sheila for she has had a nervous breakdown and both she and her daughter are now in institutions. The doctor, Dr Allin, who originally referred Sheila to us, is still in practice here in Birmingham, but I am sorry to say that it was only yesterday that he was first made aware of the chain of events which he set in motion when he asked Mrs Jones to bring Sheila to see us over 11 years ago and he is still unaware of the fact that she was a phenylketonuric, nor does he realise what the disease 'phenylketonuria' means.

The three of us are glad to say that this occasion has brought so much pleasure to our many medical colleagues not only in this country but also in Germany, in Canada and in the States, and of course last but not least, we are glad that it has brought honour to the Children's hospital here in Birmingham, to the university and to the Association of Clinical Biochemists. I do not expect that John Scott, when he made his original bequest to the City of Philadelphia in 1816, ever expected that the bestowal of his award would set in motion so many ever widening ripples of happiness, but so it is, and our happiness has made you happy and your happiness has naturally added to our own. I think it is true today, however, that the award holds a different significance for each of us; Dr Hickman thoughts are not quite the same as Horst's, nor are Horst's quite the same as mine, though both Horst and I are in full agreement with Dr Hubble in suggesting Dr Hickmans is worth 50 of us.

Just 40 years ago, strange to relate, Dr Hickmans was working, as I am today, in a university in Canada; she was lecturing in applied chemistry and dietetics at the University of Toronto. The following summer, back in England for a vacation, she received a letter from a cousin intimately concerned with the care of children asking her to see him. This she did, on the very same day. And Dr Parsons, Dr Parsons senior, for that was who her cousin was, said that she had come, not only to answer his letter, but also in answer to a prayer. She was soon installed in the clinical room by ward 6, and it was here that the biochemical department first took root. Were Sir Leonard, as we now call Dr Parsons senior, to have been here this evening he would undoubtedly, have been the first to have acknowledged his indebtedness to Dr Hickmans, for the vital role in nearly all his work. She also played a vital role in the case and management of nearly all sick children and this was recognised by the hospital when she retired a few years ago. The present occasion however affords more than local recognition, for the award, particularly as it comes from another country, ensures a niche for her in the international field, and as long as there are Phenylketonurics to be treated, the name of Dr Hickmans will be coupled with their care and management.

To Horst and myself the evening has a different significance, and here, if I may I would like to recapitulate a little. Had any one of you, sometime between 1935 and 1938 gained entry to one of the most exclusive of the ladies' colleges at Oxford, Lady Margaret Hall to be precise, you would have found there two girls of special significance to this evening. One was my wife, who captured me by pretending to fall in love with someone else- a ruse I did not see through at the time-and the other was Stella, also an expert in male psychology. At Oxford Stella was actually the first to titivate the appetite of a very famous Paediatrician present here tonight, namely Dr Benjamin Wood. She then retired for a holiday on the Adriatic coast. Here she hired a deck chair on which to recline into the sunshine. Having hired the chair she retired for a moment or two, I think, only to fetch a book, but on returning she found a German, Horst Bickel, firmly entrenched on her chair. The Germans, you may recall, at that time did not have sufficient lebensraum as they called it in their own country. Stella, being a women of character, and the Germans then being no friends of ours, ticked Horst off in no uncertain terms, and in his own vernacular, and in this way triggered off a romance which survived the tumult of war. During the war Horst's activities were confined to looking after naval personnel on land, for being colour blind he was not allowed to go to sea. As soon as the war was over Stella joined the Red Cross and, returned to Germany, ferreted Horst out. She found that he had languished in her absence-as all true lovers should-she took him to a chalet high up in the mountains in Switzerland where she restored him to health. We might interject at this point that Horst and Stella were the first proponents of the European Common Market. Having recuperated, Horst worked with Fanconi and he worked most wisely, if you know Fanconi, on the Fanconi Syndrome, and then he, in his turn, was drawn to Birmingham-Stella knew a member of the university medical staff, and it was through him that Horst was introduced to Sir Leonard Parsons who took him under his wing. By great good fortune Sir Leonard had just seen in his consultation rooms a child with Fanconi Syndrome, this diagnosis having been missed, to our delight but not surprise, by our friends in Newcastle. This child was naturally the first one to be studied by Horst in Birmingham. Here Horst turned out a great deal of original work, culminating in the preparation of the phenylalanine free formula. Those of you who were present at the International Paediatric Meeting in Montreal in 1959 will not forget the acclaim which he received from the whole of the conference at that time, yet, strange to say, when he had left Birmingham, a few years before, to return to Germany, the value of the dietary treatment of phenylketonuria being still in doubt, his contribution to Paediatrics in general and to Phenylketonuria in particular was not fully appreciated locally here. The present occasion, and the presentation of this award, has made it possible for you not only to bring him back to Birmingham, but also to tell him in no uncertain terms that he is a prophet who is greatly honoured in his own country – his own country being Birmingham.

Here I would like to digress for a few minutes to emphasize that in the preparation of the phenylalanine free formula, though now carried out commercially was no mean achievement. At the close of the meeting in Montreal, three years ago, Horst, Stella and I were taken for a wild and terrifying drive through the White Mountains, to Portland in Maine, by a figure well known to you, called Heinrich Barr. The latter had his inevitable crash, fortunately for us, two days after we had gotten out of his car. While in Portland Horst and I had the great privilege of spending an evening with Dr Földing, the discoverer of phenylketonuria. Földing was then 71, and was on his first trip to the New World. Dr Jervis, who first identified the missing enzyme in the liver of a phenylketonuric was also present, as was Mrs Földing and Stella. We were the guests of a young American paediatrician, Bill Centerwell, who, more than anyone else in the States has stressed the importance of the early detection and treatment of the phenylketonuric infant. Across the road from us was the house in which Harriet Beecher Stowe had written Uncle Tom's Cabin. During the course of the evening Dr Földing described his original studies and how he had had to obtain 20 litres of urine from his two phenylketonurics in order to have sufficient to determine the nature of the substance which turned green with the addition of ferric chloride, Horst then described how he and Dr Hickmans became as black as coalminers as they prepared the formula, using activated charcoal. Jervis then went on the say that they had discussed the dietary treatment of phenylketonuria with Block in 1940 and 1941, and that Block had said it would certainly be possible to prepare a suitable formula – or food – using activated charcoal, but when later confronted with the news that his had actually been done in Birmingham, he said that though he knew it had been theoretically possible he had always thought it would have been quite impracticable. But Dr Hickmans and Dr Bickel had done it here in Birmingham.

For myself I am sorry to say that though no award would alter my status either in Birmingham or on the other side of the Atlantic, among my friends in the States, or in Canada as a whole, in the less sophisticated world of Saskatoon, from which I come this does not apply. This is, I think, the first real honour which has come to our new medical school, and though the honour is in a way vicarious, it is nevertheless real, and has caused my colleagues and lay-personnel as well to view Paediatrics and the

Appendix V

Paediatric Department in a new light. I think it has also emphasized this fact, and this needs emphasising in a province where politics and medicine are closely interwoven, that it is only the pursuit of truth that bringeth the true glory.

In conclusion I would like to add that I too was drawn to Birmingham by Sir Leonard Parsons, but it was the restless spirit of enquiry here at that time which catalized our work. Today we are all delighted that you now have a Hubble, in the saddle, bubbling over with new ideas and catalyzing new work, as well as drawing scientifically minded people in Birmingham from all corners of the globe.

I would like to end by saying that the three of us would like to couple our thanks to you this evening with this wish, that those now working at the Children's hospital may be as richly rewarded in their turn as we have been in ours.

The 25th Anniversary Meeting of the John Scott Award – 1987

1. Scientific Meeting, Birmingham Children's Hospital
a) Birmingham Children's Hospital, 1987. *Jubilee Meeting October 24th 1987. List of Attendees.* [list] Birmingham: BCH Archive.
b) Birmingham Children's Hospital, 1987. *Jubilee Meeting October 24th 1987. Scientific Meeting Programme.* [programme] Birmingham: BCH Archive.

2. Evening Celebrations at Birmingham Botanical Gardens
a) Reunion Dinner, 1987. The Botanical Gardens, Birmingham: BCH Archive.

3. Letters and Notes
a) Gerrard, J., 1987. *Letter to Anne Green about John Scott Award.* [letter] (Personal communication 6 December 1987). Birmingham: BCH Archive.
b) Mann, S and McKeown, C., 1987. *Jubilee Meeting October 24th 1987. Resumes of the Scientific Meeting.* [notes] Birmingham: BCH Archive.

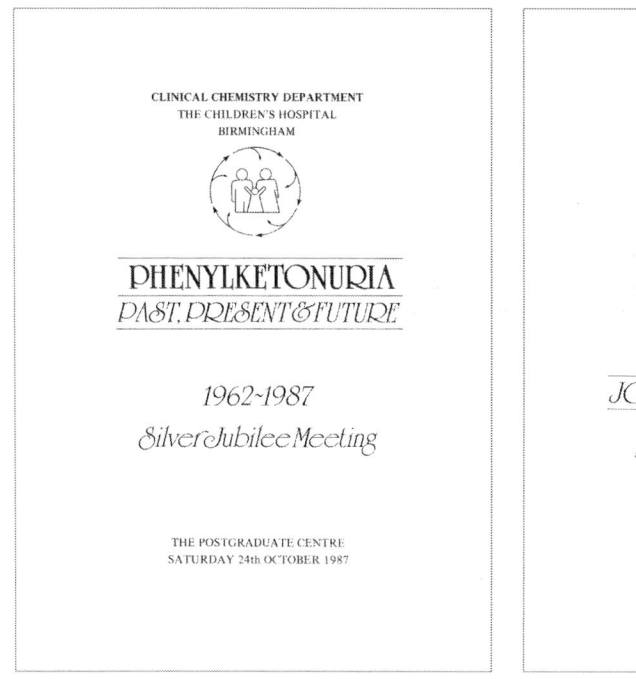

1b) Scientific programme.

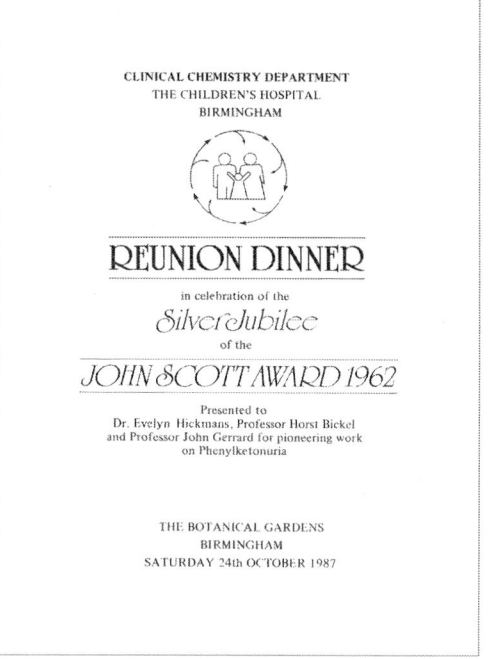

2a) Reunion Dinner.

PERSONAL REFLECTIONS BY THE AUTHOR

This has been a personal journey for me as we reflect on Sheila's life and legacy.

When I came to Birmingham in 1968 to do an MSc at Birmingham University, I had never heard of PKU and inherited metabolic disorders (IMD) were in their infancy. Newborn screening was barely in existence. My introduction to Clinical Chemistry was to establish a method for measuring methylmalonic acid (MMA) in urine as an indicator of vitamin B12 deficiency; this was in the Biochemistry laboratories at the former General Hospital, now the Children's Hospital on Steelhouse Lane. Little did I know I would come full circle by working in the same building 30 years later when I retired. I also didn't know at the time how important MMA would become in the field of IMD.

Serendipity took its course when I got a job in 1971 at BCH, at Ladywood, as a junior biochemist working with the late Dr Noel Raine. This was a baptism of fire and I was soon introduced to newborn screening and performing the PKU screening for babies born in the city of Birmingham became part of my routine daily work. Indeed, a positive screen result caused great excitement for the laboratory staff just as it must have done for Dr Bickel and Dr Hickmans with the ferric chloride test. Another one of my jobs was to perform paper chromatography of amino acids on plasma and urine specimens using the large glass tanks that I feel certain were the same ones used by Dr Hickmans and Dr Bickel. I remember the overwhelming smell of the noxious solvents in this small room (still no fume cupboards in those days!), when I took the papers out for drying, and the almost permanent purple staining of my fingers.

During those early days I became aware of the important history of PKU from within the department but never once considered that I might meet Sheila Jones as no one knew what had happened to her. I was initially at BCH for five years which made a big impression, I loved the work, and it set my destiny as a Paediatric Biochemist. I had a six year spell at Sheffield Children's Hospital where I was fortunate to get to know and collaborate with Rodney Pollitt and continue my interest in IMD. I came back to BCH to Head the Department in 1982 after the untimely death of Noel Raine, from whom I had learnt a great deal. When I arrived at my 'new' office I remember finding a large glass column covered with dust on the windowsill. Noel Raine had told me about this so I knew what it was: the column used to prepare the first diet for PKU. Determined it should be given a place of honour – it was housed in a special purpose-built cabinet (courtesy of Scientific Hospital Supplies) and subsequently moved with the department to the new Children's Hospital in 1998. Noel Raine was a hoarder par excellence and I too developed this tendency, so between us the important memorabilia and historical documentation about Sheila, which is now able to archived, had been kept for almost 70 years.

My career has been intertwined with the Sheila Jones story on different occasions. Confirming the diagnosis of PKU and then meeting Sheila in 1987 was a significant moment for me as were her final years at Chelmsley Hospital and her subsequent funeral. There was a sadness that no-one knew anything about her life or her family and certain assumptions had been made which were not true. Interestingly it seems likely that I unknowingly had met Sheila's brother, Trevor and his wife, Marilyn, when they came to BCH for PKU carrier testing in the 1970s as this was one of my early jobs at BCH.

I had the privilege to meet Horst Bickel at numerous scientific events and welcomed him and John Gerrard to Birmingham for the 1987 celebration of the John Scott Award. More recently I have subsequently been able to make contact with both of their families in Germany and Canada respectively. Sadly, I never met Evelyn Hickmans nor have been able to trace any of her wider family.

This book has been on my 'to do' list longer than I want to admit. The main catalyst for writing it was undoubtedly the honour of giving the Stuart Green Memorial Lecture in June 2017 at BCH. Stuart, a Paediatric Neurologist with a keen interest in IMD, was a dear friend and colleague at BCH who welcomed me as a scientist into his clinical team in the early 1980s. For me this opportunity illustrated the value of scientists and medical doctors working together for the benefit of patients and their families, just as Evelyn Hickmans, Horst Bickel and John Gerrard had done in 1951.

As I got to know more about Sheila's life I became determined to preserve the historical documents and to write this story so others could know about it. Soon after I had started in earnest to write this book (August 2017) I had a major setback with a back injury which lead to surgery. It took its toll for many months whilst I was supported by my dear husband Richard and several special friends and family. Some months later I decided to re-visit my very early draft and use my enforced confinement at home to try to do some writing. It was extremely difficult at first – only 10 minutes sitting down at the computer each time but it proved to be the catalyst to slowly continue on to the finish. As I slowly improved (April 2018), and with one of the hottest summers in England, I resumed work in earnest.

Personal Reflections by the Author

For a scientist used to a logical approach, with hypothesis, experiment, results and conclusions as a format for publications, this has been a unique departure from my other writings and a big challenge. The business of other people's lives and writing a story is a tricky one which does not come naturally to me. I owe a huge amount to all those who have helped me but especially Sheila's brothers and in particular Trevor. I was made most welcome at his home and it has been a privilege and pleasure to get to know Sheila's family and be able to write this story in her memory. The friendship and understanding developed with her family has been a reward for me I could not have ever imagined. If I have inadvertently caused any intrusion in their lives, I hope it has had some benefits for them too.

There is never an end point when writing as there is always more to find out and more to do, but one has to draw a line which I did at the end of 2019. BUT – COVID-19 then unexpectedly interrupted the final stages of the work as we were confined to our homes – but with a bit of innovation, collaboration and the wonders of technology we got there. A special thank you goes to all those who helped through this exceptional time. Of course I would be delighted to hear of any new information which others are aware of or I have inadvertently omitted or misrepresented. I hope you have enjoyed reading the story.

Anne Green

'There is no education like adversity.'
(Benjamin Disraeli)

BIBLIOGRAPHY and REFERENCES

The author is grateful to the Library and Knowledge Service at Birmingham Women's and Children's NHS Foundation Trust, for help sourcing and collating references, and seeking copyright permissions, with special thanks to Ann Daly, Library Manager. The listing below includes specific published references, some archived documents (not listed elsewhere in this publication) and general background reading. All material is grouped into sections.

Enquiries about material in the BCH Archive should be directed to the Library Manager at *bwc.library@nhs.net*.

HISTORY OF BIRMINGHAM

Birmingham City Council, 2011. *Population and Census*. [online] Available at: *https://www.birmingham.gov.uk/info/20057/about_birmingham/1294/population_and_census*.

Caswell, P., 1997. *Kings Norton*. Stroud: Tempus Publishing.

Chinn, C., 2013. *Carl Chinn: No-frills living in city back-to-backs*. [online] Available at: *https://www.birminghammail.co.uk/news/nostalgia/carl-chinn-no-frills-living-in-city-403144*.

Lambert, T., 2019. *A Brief History of Birmingham, England*. [online] Available at: *http://www.localhistories.org/birmingham.html*.

Muckross House Research Library, n.d. *Ireland in the 1930s-1940s*. [online] Available at: *http://www.muckrosshouseresearchlibrary.ie/Ireland-1930s-1940s.php*.

National Trust, n.d. *Birmingham Back to Backs*. [online] Available at: *https://www.nationaltrust.org.uk/birmingham-back-to-backs*.

Pearson, W., 2004. *Kings Norton Past and Present*. Stroud: Sutton Publishing.

Rudge, T. and Joseph, M., 2015. *Birmingham: We Lived Back to Back – The Real Story*. Oxford: Fronthill Media.

Stephens, W.B., 1964. The Growth of the City. In: W.B. Stephens [ed.], 1964. *A History of the County of Warwick: Volume 7, the City of Birmingham*. London: Victoria County Hospital, pp.4-25. Available at: *https://www.british-history.ac.uk/vch/warks/vol7/pp4-25*.

Wikipedia, 2019. *Birmingham Union Workhouse*. [online] Available at: *https://en.wikipedia.org/wiki/Birmingham_Union_Workhouse*.

Bibliography and References

BIRMINGHAM HOSPITALS
Lordswood Maternity Hospital (44 Lordswood Road)
The Harborne Society, 2014. Lordswood Maternity Hospital: Brief History of the Property. *The Harborne Society Newsletter*, 82, pp.6-7.
Lordswood Nursery Ladies Sub-committee, 1928-30. *Lordswood Nursery Ladies Sub-committee Minutes*. [minutes]. Birmingham Poor Law Union. GP B/2/6/14. Birmingham: Archives and Heritage.

East Birmingham's Hospitals 1895-1995
Ayres, J.G., Ellis, C.J. and Portsmouth, O.H.D., 1995. *East Birmingham's Hospitals, 1895-1995: from City Hospital, Little Bromwich, to Birmingham Heartlands Hospital*. Aldridge: Norman A. Tector.

Highcroft Hall Hospital
Baker, C. 2007. Highcroft Hall Hospital. [online]. Extracted from: M.Hinson [ed.], 2001. *Highcroft: From Workhouse to Modern Mental Health Service*. Birmingham: Highcroft History Group. Available at: *http://bhamb14.co.uk/index-files/HIGHCROFTHALLHOSPITAL.htm*.

Chelmsley Hospital
Jumbo GB, n.d. *History*. [online] Available at: *http://www.jumbogb.org.uk/PAGES/historypage.htm*.

General Hospital / University Medical School
Wikipedia, 2019. *Birmingham General Hospital*. [online] Available at: *https://en.wikipedia.org/wiki/Birmingham_General_Hospital*.
University of Birmingham, n.d. *History of the University of Birmingham Medical School, 1825-2001*. [online] Available at: *https://www.birmingham.ac.uk/university/colleges/mds/about/history.aspx*.

BIRMINGHAM CHILDREN'S HOSPITAL
Birmingham Children's Hospital Charity, n.d. *Our History*. [online] Available at: *https://www.bch.org.uk/pages/faqs/category/history*.
Birmingham Children's Hospital Charity, n.d. *A History of Birmingham Children's Hospital*. [manuscript] Birmingham: BCH Archive.
Rimmer, D., 1999. *The Diana Princess of Wales Children's Hospital, Birmingham 1862-1999*. London: Assorted Images.
Waterhouse, R., 1962. *Children in Hospital: A Hundred Years of Child Care in Birmingham*. London: Hutchinson.

Leonard G. Parsons

Brown, G.H. n.d., *Leonard Gregory (Sir) Parsons.* [online] Available at: *https://history.rcplondon.ac.uk/inspiring-physicians/leonard-gregory-sir-parsons.*

Dunn, P.M., 2002. Sir Leonard Parsons of Birmingham (1879-1950) and antenatal paediatrics. *Archives of Disease in Childhood. Fetal and Neonatal Edition,* 86(1), pp.F65-7.

Parsons, L., 1910-1951. *University of Birmingham Staff Papers: Papers of Sir Leonard Parsons Collection.* [collection] GB 150 US48. Birmingham: University of Birmingham, Cadbury Research Library, Special Collections.

University of Birmingham, n.d. *History of the Medical School.* [online] Available at: *https://www.birmingham.ac.uk/schools/medical-school/about/history.aspx.*

James M. Smellie

Anon, 1961. J.M. Smellie, O.B.E, M.D., F.R.C.P. *British Medical Journal,* 1(5232), pp.1113-4.

John W. Gerrard

Family of J. Gerrard, 2019. *John Gerrard.* [letters] (Personal communications, 2019). Birmingham: BCH Archive.

Gerrard, J.W., 1985. *Accepting the Ross Award.* [speech] (Delivered September 9 1985). Transcript available from Birmingham: BCH Archive.

Rosenberg, A. n.d. *John Watson Gerrard.* [online] Available at: *https://history.rcplondon.ac.uk/inspiring-physicians/john-watson-gerrard.*

The Saskatoon StarPhoenix, 2013. John Gerrard, Obituary. *The Saskatoon StarPhoenix.* 5 March, p.4c.

Evelyn M. Hickmans

Broughton, P. and Lines, J., 1996. *The Association of Clinical Biochemists: First Forty Years.* London: ACB Venture Publications.

Cant, W. 1972. Dr Evelyn Hickmans – Biochemistry and Paediatrics. *The Times,* 58391, p.16.

Raine, D.N., 1972. Evelyn Marion Hickmans. *Lancet,* 299(7745), pp.331-2.

Rayner-Canham, M. and Rayer-Canham, G., 2008. *Chemistry was their life: Pioneer British Women Chemists, 1880-1949.* London: Imperial College Press.

Horst Bickel

Bickel, H., 1952. *Aminoaciduria in Childhood.* PhD. University of Birmingham.

Family of Bickel, H., 2019. *Horst Bickel.* [letters] (Personal communications 2019). Birmingham: BCH Archive.

Hoffmann, G. F., 2001. In Memoria Horst Bickel. *Journal of Inherited Metabolic Disease,* 24, pp.611-3.

Hoffman, G., 2001. *In Memoriam Univ.-Prof. Dr. med. Dr. h.c. Horst Bickel, Ph.D., F.R.C.P.* [speech] (Delivered at conference in 2001). Transcript available from Birmingham: BCH Archive.

Liberra, M., 2015. *Michael Liberra (Bickel) – E.S.PKU Conference 2015.* [video online] Available at: *https://www.youtube.com/watch?v=nNp_HUrGu-c.*

Osten, P., 2015. Horst Bickel und der Weg zur Therapie der Phenylketonurie. In: G. F. Hoffmann, W. Eckart, and P. Osten (eds.), 2015. *Entwicklungen und Perspektiven der Kinder-und Jugendmedizin, 150 Jahre Pädiatrie.* Heidelberg: Universitätsklinikum Heidelberg, pp.139-69.

Royal College of Physicians, n.d. *Horst Bickel.* [online] Available at: *https://history.rcplondon.ac.uk/inspiring-physicians/horst-bickel.*

Trefz, F., Buist, N. and The Members of the Society for Inherited Metabolic Disorders, 2001. In Memoriam: Horst Bickel (1918-2000). *Molecular Genetics and Metabolism,* 72(4), pp.277-8.

LEARNING DISABILITY SERVICES IN THE UK

County Asylums, n.d. *The History of the Asylum.* [online] Available at: *https://www.countyasylums.co.uk/history/.*

Higginbottom, P., n.d. *Birmingham, Warwickshire.* [online] Available at: *http://www.workhouses.org.uk/Birmingham/.*

Killaspy, H., 2006. From the asylum to community care: learning from experience. *British Medical Bulletin,* 79-80(1), pp.245-58.

Open University, n.d. *Timeline of learning disability history.* [online] Available at: *http://www.open.ac.uk/health-and-social-care/research/shld/timeline-learning-disability-history.*

Roberts, A., 2019. *Mental Health History Timeline.* [online] Available at: *http://studymore.org.uk/mhhtim.htm.*

Turner, J., Hayward, R., Angel, K., Fulford, B., Hall, J., Millard, C. and Thomson, M., 2015. The History of Mental Health Services in Modern England: Practitioner Memories and the Direction of Future Research. *Medical History,* 59(4), pp.599-624.

Wikipedia, 2019. *Care in the Community.* [online] Available at: *https://en.wikipedia.org/wiki/Care_in_the_Community.*

HISTORY OF PHENYLKETONURIA

Alonsso-Fernandez, J.R., 2009. The contributions of Louis I Woolf to the treatment, early diagnosis and understanding of phenylketonuria. *Journal of Medical Screening,* 16(4), pp.205-11.

Buck, P., 1950. *The Child Who Never Grew.* New York: The John Day Company.

Følling, A.,1934. Über Ausscheidung von Phenylbrenztraubensäure in den Harn als Stoffwechselanomalie in Verbindung mit Imbezillität (The excretion of phenylpyruvic acid in the urine, an anomaly of metabolism in connection with imbecility). *Zeitschrift für physiologische Chemie,* 227, pp.169-176. Translated from German by S.H. Boyer, 1963. In: P.S. Harper (ed.), 2004. *Landmarks in Medical Genetics: Classic Papers with Commentaries.* Oxford: Oxford University Press, pp.23-6.

Gonzalez, J. and Willis, M.S., 2010. Ivar Asbjörn Følling: Discovered Phenylketonuria (PKU). *Laboratory Medicine,* 41(2), pp.118-9.

Güttler, F., 1984. Phenylketonuria: 50 years since Følling's Discovery and still Expanding our Clinical and Biochemical Knowledge. *Acta Paediatrica Scandinavia,* 73(6), pp.705-26.

Jervis, G.A., 1953. Phenylpyruvic oligophrenia: deficiency of phenylalanine oxidising system. *Proceedings of the Society for Experimental Biology and Medicine,* 82(3), p.514-5.

Koch, J., 1997. *Robert Guthrie: The PKU Story.* Pasadena: Hope Publishing House. (Kindly provided to the author as a gift from friend and colleague Jim Bonham).

Messner, D.A., 2012. *On the Scent: The Discovery of PKU.* [online] Available at: *https://www.sciencehistory.org/distillations/on-the-scent-the-discovery-of-pku.*

Munro, T.A., 1947. Phenylketonuria: Data on Forty-Seven British Families. *Annals of Eugenics,* 14, pp.60-88.

Paul, D.B. and Brosco, J., 2013. *The PKU Paradox: A Short History of a Genetic Disease.* Baltimore: John Hopkins University Press.

Penrose, L.S., 1938. *A Clinical and Genetic Study of 1,280 Cases of Mental Defect.* London: His Majesty's Stationery Office.

Penrose, L.S., 1946. Phenylketonuria: A Problem in Eugenics. *Lancet,* 2407(6409), pp.949-53.

Woolf, L.I. and Vulliamy, D.G., 1951. Phenylketonuria with a study of the effect upon it of glutamic acid. *Archives of Disease in Childhood,* 26(130), pp.487-94.

SHEILA – DIAGNOSIS AND TREATMENT

Bickel, H., 1952. *Aminoaciduria in Childhood*. PhD. University of Birmingham.

Bickel, H., Gerrard, J. and Hickmans, E.M., 1953. Influence of Phenylalanine intake on Phenylketonuria. *Lancet*, 265(6790), pp.812-3.

Bickel, H., Gerrard, J. and Hickmans, E.M., 1954. The Influence of Phenylalanine Intake on the Chemistry and Behaviour of a Phenylketonuria Child. *Acta Paediatrica*, 43(1), pp.64-77.

Bickel, H., 1954. The Effects of a Phenylalanine-Free and Phenylalanine-Poor Diet in Phenylpyruvic Oligophrenia. *Experimental Medicine and Surgery*, 12(1-2), pp.114-8.

Bickel, H., 1996. The first treatment of phenylketonuria. *European Journal of Pediatrics*, 155(Suppl. 1), pp.s.2-3.

Blainey, J.D. and Gulliford, R., 1956. Phenylalanine-restricted Diets in the Treatment of Phenylketonuria. *Archives of Disease in Childhood*, 31(160), pp.452-66.

Block, R.J. and Bolling, D., 1951. *The amino acid composition of proteins and foods: analytical methods and results*. 2nd ed. Springfield: Charles C. Thomas.

E.S.PKU, 2018. *The legacy of Professor Horst Bickel*. [video online] Available at: *https://youtu.be/VMBAsk367ok*.

Gerrard, J.W., n.d. *Sheila Jones*. [clinical notes] Birmingham: BCH Archive.

Gerrard, J.W., 1994. Phenylketonuria revisited. *Clinical and Investigative Medicine*, 17(5), pp.510-3.

Henderson, L.M. and Snell, E.S., 1948. A Uniform Medium for Determinations of Amino Acids with Various Microorganisms. *Journal of Biologic Chemistry*, 172(1), pp.15-29.

Penrose, L. and Quastel, J.H., 1937. Metabolic Studies in Phenylketonuria. *The Biochemical Journal*, 31(2), pp.266-74.

Phenylketonuria: The Early Years, 2008. [compilation of films, including film from H. Bickel, 1952] Edited by A. Green. Birmingham: BCH Archive.

Schramm, G. and Primosigh, J., 1943. Über die quantitative Trennung neutraler Aminosäuren durch Chromatographie. *Berichte der Deutschen Chemischen Gesellschaft*, 76(4), pp.373-86.

Tiselius, A., 1947. Adsorption Analysis of Amino Acid Mixtures. In M.L. Anson and J.T. Edsall (eds.), 1947. *Advances in Protein Chemistry*. Cambridge: Academic Press, pp.67-93.

PKU EARLY DEVELOPMENTS – DIET AND TREATMENT

Armstrong, J.A. and Tyler, F.H., 1955. Studies on phenylketonuria I. Restricted phenylalanine intake in phenylketonuria. *The Journal of Clinical Investigation,* 34(4), pp.565-80.

Blainey, J. D. and Squire, J. R., 1960. The Management and Diagnosis of Phenylketonuria. In: B.W. Richards (ed.), 1962. *Proceedings of the London Conference on the Scientific Study of Mental Deficiency.* Dagenham: May & Baker, pp.119-25.

Blainey J.D. and Leyton G.B., 1963. Balance Studies in Phenylketonuria. *Journal of Mental Deficiency Research,* 7(1), pp.22-30.

Bickel, H. and Grueter, W., 1960. The Dietary Treatment of Phenylketonuria: Experiences During the Past 9 Years. In P.W. Bowman and H.V. Mautner (eds.), 1960. *Proceedings of the First International Conference of Mental Retardation.* New York: Grune and Stratton, pp.272-6.

Birch, H.G. and Tizard, J., 1967. The Dietary Treatment of Phenylketonuria: Not Proven. *Developmental Medicine and Child Neurology,* 9(1), pp.9-12.

Brimblecombe, F.S.W., Blainey, J.D., Stoneman, M.E.R. and Wood, B.S.B., 1961. Dietary and Biochemical Control of Phenylketonuria. *British Medical Journal,* 2(5255), pp.793-8.

Clothier, C., 2019. *Memoirs.* [Unpublished]. Birmingham: BCH Archive.

Smith, I., Lobascher, M.E., Stevenson, J.E., Wolff, O.H., Schmidt, H., Gruber-Kaiser, S. and Bickel, H., 1978. Effect of stopping low-phenylalanine diet on intellectual progress of children with phenylketonuria. *British Medical Journal,* 2(6139), pp.723-6.

Wikipedia, 2019. *SHS International.* [online] Available at: *https://en.wikipedia.org/wiki/SHS_International.*

Williams (formerly Griffiths), P., 1954. *Letter from Allen and Hanburys to Chief Dietitian, Bristol Royal Hospital for Sick Children.* [letter] (Personal communication, August 23 1954). Birmingham: BCH Archive.

Woolf, L.I., Griffiths, R. and Moncrieff, A., 1955. Treatment of Phenylketonuria with a diet low in Phenylalanine. *British Medical Journal,* 1(4905), pp.57-64.

Woolf, L.I., Griffiths, R., Moncrieff, A., Coates, S. and Dillstone, F., 1958. The Dietary Treatment of Phenylketonuria. *Archives of Disease in Childhood,* 33(167), pp.31-45.

Woolf, L.I., 1963. Inherited Metabolic Disorders: Errors of phenylalanine and tyrosine. *Advances in Clinical Chemistry,* 6, pp.97-230.

Woolf, L.I., 1967. The Dietary Treatment of Phenylketonuria: not proven. *Developmental Medicine in Child Neurology,* 9(2), pp.244-5.

PKU – NEWBORN SCREENING

Armstrong, M.D. and Binkley, E.L., 1956. Studies on phenylketonuria. V. Observations on a newborn infant with phenylketonuria. *Proceedings of the Society for Experimental Biology and Medicine*, 93(3), pp.418-20.

Bickel, H., 1980. Phenylketonuria: Past, present, future. *Journal of Inherited Metabolic Disease*, 3(1), pp.123-32.

Boyd, M.M.M., 1961. Phenylketonuria: City of Birmingham Screening Survey. *British Medical Journal*, 1(5228), pp.771-3.

The Consultant Paediatricians and Medical Officers of Health of the S.E. Scotland Hospital Region, 1968. Population screening by Guthrie test for phenylketonuria in South-east Scotland. *British Medical Journal*, 1(5593), pp.674-6.

Department of Health and Social Security, 1967-1969. *Screening for early detection of Phenylketonuria.* [policy] MH 159/39. Ministry of Health and Department of Health and Social Security. London: The National Archives, Kew.

Downing, M. and Pollitt, R., 2008. Newborn bloodspot screening in the UK – past, present and future. *Annals of Clinical Biochemistry*, 45(1), pp.11-7.

E.S.PKU, n.d. *Who we are.* [online] Available at: *https://www.espku.org/who-we-are*.

Gibbs, N.K. and Woolf, L.I., 1959. Tests for Phenylketonuria. *British Medical Journal*, 2(5151), pp.532-5.

Griffith, S.P., Morris, J., Assheton, J. and Green, A., 1987. An On-Line Computerized System for Neonatal Screening. In: B.L.Therrall [ed.], 1987. *Advances in Neonatal Screening*. Amsterdam: Elsevier Science Publishers pp.513-6.

Guthrie, R. and Susi, A., 1963. A simple phenylalanine method for detecting Phenylketonuria in large populations of newborn infants. *Pediatrics*, 32, pp.338-43.

Mahon, D.F., 1973. Scriver Testing for Inherited Metabolic Diseases. *Nursing Mirror*, 137(2), pp.10-5.

Medical Research Council of the Conference on Phenylketonuria, 1963. Treatment of Phenylketonuria. *British Medical Journal*, 1(5347), pp.1691-7.

Medical Research Council Steering Committee for the MRC/DHSS Phenylketonuria Register, 1981. Routine Neonatal Screening for Phenylketonuria in the United Kingdom 1964-78. *British Medical Journal (Clinical Research Edition)*, 282(6277), pp.1680-4.

Medical Research Council Working Party on Phenylketonuria, 1968. Present status of different mass screening procedures for phenylketonuria. *British Medical Journal*, 4(5622), pp.7-13.

Medical Research Council Working Party on Phenylketonuria, 1993. Recommendations on the dietary management of Phenylketonuria. *Archives of Disease in Childhood,* 68(3), pp.426-7.

Medical Research Council Working Party on Phenylketonuria, 1993. Phenylketonuria due to phenylalanine hydroxylase deficiency: an unfolding story. *BMJ,* 306(6830), pp.115-9.

NSPKU, n.d. *History.* [online] Available at: *https://www.nspku.org/history-of-nspku/*.

Scriver, C.R., Davies, E., Cullen, A.M., 1964. Application of a simple micromethod to the screening of plasma for a variety of aminoacidopathies. *The Lancet,* 284(7353), pp.230-2.

Smith, I., Cook, B. and Beasley, M., 1991. Review of Neonatal Screening Programme for Phenylketonuria. *BMJ,* 303(6798), pp.333-5.

Welsh Hospital Board, 1968-1970. *Screening for early detection of Phenylketonuria.* [policy] BD 18/737. Welsh Hospital Board. London: The National Archives, Kew.

Woolf, L.I., 1967. Large scale screening for metabolic diseases in the newborn in Great Britain. In J.A. Anderson and K.F. Swaiman, 1967. *Phenylketonuria and Allied Metabolic Diseases.* Washington: U.S. Department of Health, Education, and Welfare, Social and Rehabilitation Service, Children's Bureau, pp.50-61.

Woolf, L.I., 1968. Mass Screening of the Newborn for Metabolic Disease. *Archives of Disease in Childhood,* 43, pp.137-140.

JOHN SCOTT AWARD

Annals of Clinical Biochemistry, 1963. The John Scott Award: The Presentation of the John Scott Award for 1962 to Dr. Evelyn M. Hickmans. *Annals of Clinical Biochemistry,* 2(5), pp.106-8.

Birmingham Post, 1962. Awards for Medical Research Workers. 24.10.1962

City of Philadelphia, 2018. *The John Scott Award Recipients.* [online] Available at: *http://www.garfield.library.upenn.edu/johnscottaward/johnscottaward%28full%29.html*.

Fox, R., 1968. The John Scott Medal. *Proceedings of the American Philosophical Society,* 112(6), pp.416-30.

Wikipedia, 2018. *Cuban Missile Crisis.* [online] Available at: *https://en.wikipedia.org/wiki/Cuban_Missile_Crisis.*

Wikipedia, 2019. *John Scott Medal.* [online] Available at: *https://en.wikipedia.org/wiki/John_Scott_Medal.*

SHEILA JONES AWARD

E.S.PKU, 2019. *Sheila Jones Award*. [online] Available at: https://www.espku.org/sheila-jones-award/.

Muresan, I.B., 2018. *LAURA PETREUȘ– Recunoaștere internațională pentru o luptătoare, vreme de 15 ani, pentru PKU!* [online] Available at: http://www.graiul.ro/2018/11/15/laura-petreus-recunoastere-internationala-pentru-o-luptatoare-vreme-de-15-ani-pentru-pku/.

PKU TODAY

Blau, N., 2016. Genetics of Phenylketonuria: Then and Now. *Human Mutation*, 37(6), pp.508-15.

Isabella, V.M., Ha, B.N., Castillo, M.J., Lubkowicz, D.J., Rowe, S.E., Millet, Y.A., Anderson, C.L., Li, N., Fisher, A.B., West, K.A., Reeder, P.J., Momin, M.M., Bergeron, C.G., Guilmain, S.E., Miller, P.F., Kurtz, C.B., Falb, D., 2018. Development of a synthetic live bacterial therapeutic for the human metabolic disease phenylketonuria. *Nature Biotechnology*, 36, pp.857-64.

Lichter-Konecki, U. and Vockley, J., 2019. Phenylketonuria: Current Treatments and Future Developments. *Drugs*, 79, pp.495-500.

Longo, N., Dimmock, D., Levy, H., Viau, K., Bausell, H., Bilder, D.A., Burton, B., Gross, C., Northrup, H., Roher, F., Sacharow, S., Sanchez-Valle, A., Stuy, M., Thomas, J., Vockley, J., Zori, R. and Harding, C.O., 2019. Evidence – and consensus-based recommendations for the use of pegvaliase in adults with phenylketonuria. *Genetics in Medicine*, 21(8), pp.1851-67.

MacDonald, A., Blau, N., 2016. Dietary Management of PKU. In: N. Blau [ed.], 2016. *Phenylketonuria and BH4 Deficiencies*. 3rd ed. Breman: Uni-Med Verlag Ag.

Muntau, A.C., du Moulin, M. and Feillet, F., 2018. Diagnostic and therapeutic recommendations for the treatment of hyperphenylalaninemia in patients 0-4 years of age. *Orphanet Journal of Rare Diseases*, 13(1), p.173.

Preece, M.A. and Goddard, P., 2019. *West Midlands Newborn Screening Annual Report 2018/2019*. [letter] (Personal communication September 2019). Birmingham: BCH Archive.

Public Health England, 2019. *Newborn blood spot screening: programme overview*. [online] Available at: https://www.gov.uk/guidance/newborn-blood-spot-screening-programme-overview.

Woo, S.L.C., Lidskey, A.S., Güttler, F., Chandra, T. and Robson, K.J.H., 1983. Cloned human phenylalanine hydroxylase gene allows prenatal diagnosis and carrier detection of classical phenylketonuria. *Nature*, 306, pp.151-5.

INDEX

Index Notes: biographical details are listed in chronological order.

Acts of Parliament 127-9
Alder Hey Children's Hospital, Liverpool 92
Allen and Hanburys 40, 55, 86
Allin, Dr. 10, 24, 59-60, 100-101, 111, 148
amino acid chromatography 17, 30-33, 41, 134, 135
   'Scriver' technique *94*, 95
   room at BCH (1970s-1980s) 32-3
aminoacidurias 17
Association of Clinical Biochemists 99, 141-3
Aston, Birmingham 61-4, 114
Austin Motor Company 1, 2-3, 123-4

back-to-back houses 62-63, 71-73, 74, 114, 124
Baines, Dr 148
Belton, Neville 100
Bickel, Horst
  amino acid chromatography work 30-3
  biographical details 14, 17-18, 33-4, 49, 149-50
  receives John Scott Award 98-102,
    attends 25th Anniversary Meeting 103
  Sheila's case 35-8, 40-4, 47-50, 51-3, 60, 80, 113
    personal notes on 135
    stills from film taken of Sheila *51, 52*
  suggests testing for PKU 24
Bickel, Stella 17, 102, 149

Biochemistry Laboratory (BCH)
  archival notes 131-5
  blood specimen collection 26-7
  history
    (1923-50) staff and tests 14-15, 28-9
    (1950s) casein hydrolysate processes 40-43, 55
    (1950s) chromatography methods 29-32, 40
    (1970s-1980s) chromatography room 32-3
  phenylalanine loading test on Trevor Jones 115
  Sheila's analysis and treatment *see* Jones, Sheila
  Sheila's special mixture
    charcoal column used 41
    discontinued 58-9
    phenylalanine challenge at home 49-50
    phenylalanine challenge observations 51-4
    pressure of production 48-9
    Winchester bottle 46
Birmingham and Midland Free Hospital for Sick Children 125-6
Birmingham Children's Hospital
  biochemistry department *see* Biochemistry Laboratory (BCH)
  blood-based newborn screening 93-5
  doctors' concerns during treatment of Sheila 48
  professional reactions to findings 54, 56

Index

Gray, Professor Sir Muir 122
history
   (1917-1950s) 11-13
   (1951) 13-18
   summary of pioneering PKU treatment 118-21
   Inherited Metabolic Disorders laboratory 80-81
   John Scott Award ceremony (1962) 99-101
   25th Anniversary Meeting 103, 152
   commemorative plaque 102
patients successfully treated 108
photographs
   Biochemistry Laboratory staff 28
   Honour board (1948-1958) 16
   John Scott Award plaque 102
   Ladywood Site (1950s) 11
   Newborn Screening Laboratory staff 117
   'Scriver' technique laboratory equipment 94
   Sheila's brothers' visit 116-17
Sheila Jones Award 104-5
   and plaque to Sheila 85
Sheila's referral to (1951) 18-19
   diagnosis and treatment *see* Jones, Sheila
   and end of Sheila's follow up 59-60
wards
   care of Sheila 42
   layout (1940s-1950s) 12
   organisation and rules (1940s-1950s) 25-6
Birmingham Family Services Unit (FSU) 71, 114
Birmingham history 123-4
   Austin Motor Company 1, 2-3, 123-4
   hospitals 125-6, 129-30
   housing 62, 124
   map (1959) *xviii-xix*

photographs
   Aston, Lichfield Road 61
   Aston, Victoria Road 61
   Austin works (1930s and 1940s) 2-3
   back-to-backs 62
   bomb damage (WWII) 3-4
   Highcroft Hall Hospital 65
   Kings Norton, The Green 5-6
   Tyseley, Matlock Road 7
   Shenley Cottage Homes 65
   United Birmingham Teaching Hospitals 13
   World War II and Irish immigration 1-2
Birmingham hospitals, history 125-6
Blainey, J.D. 55, 59, 89-90
Block, R.J. 39, 42, 150
Bristol Children's Hospital 86
Brooklands Hospital 81-3, 130
Buck, Pearl 119
Bush, I.E. 100

Chelmsley Hospital 66-85
   buildings 67, 70-1
     photographs 67-8, 70
   care routine 73-4, 75-6
     activities and outings 76-9
     photographs of staff 76
   case workers attached to 70-1, 114-15
   conditions of Sheila's admission 66, 68-70
     clinical notes 69
     mother's visits 71
   history 66-8, 129-30
     reorganisation (1990s) 81
   volunteers and helpers 76, 78
chromatography *see* amino acid chromatography
City Hospital 125
City of Philadelphia letters 137, 144-5
Clothier, Christine 87-89

Davies, Professor Dame Sally xi
Day, Tom 29-30, 32, 33-4, 103
Dent, Charles 30
dietary treatment for PKU,
   demonstrating the effects of 89-91
   diet for life 107-9
   diets and paediatric dietetics
      development 88-9
   genetics 109
   idea of, and development 38-40
   management and digital technology
      107
   national strategy (1970s) 79-80
   preparation at BCH 40-42
      handwritten notes (1964) 132-4
   protein substitutes development 86-8,
      107
      commercial products 87, *107*
      advances 88-9
dietary trials of low phenylalanine diet
   (BCH)
   corroborating studies (1950s) 54
   history and significance of 118-21
   phenylalanine challenge 49-50
      effects on patient 51-4
   phenylalanine free diet 42-3
   phenylalanine reduced diet 43-9
      during pregnancy 80
   see also dietary treatment, national
      strategy

Ear, Nose and Throat Hospital 125
Education Act (1970) 67, 129
European Medicines Agency 109
European Society for Phenylketonuria and
   Allied Disorders (E.S.PKU) 95,
   104-5
Eye Hospital 125

Family Services Unit 71, 114
Fanconi, Guido 17, 24, 149

ferric chloride testing
   early testing 21, 150
      extended to PKU 22-3
   newborn screening 91-2, 96
   of Sheila 24, 25, 43, 58, 131-2, 134
   see also phenylalanine
Finch, Ethel 29
Følling, Ivar Asbjørn 20-22, 150

genetic studies 109, 110
   inherited metabolic disorders 21-2,
      92, 153
Gerrard, Betty 103, 148-9
Gerrard, John
   dietary work 42, 55
      notes on 135
   on Evelyn Hickmans 97, 102
   professional life 13, 15-16, 54
   receives John Scott Award 98-102
      25th anniversary (1987) *103*, 154
      ceremony photographs 99, *101*
      City of Philadelphia letter 137
      medal 98
      speech (1962) 102, 147-51
   Sheila's case 18, 38, 59-60, 111
      recollections of Sheila 55, 100-101
Gerrard, Jon 102
Gilding, Peter 29
Gray, Muir 122
Great Ormond Street Hospital 40, 54, 87
Green, Anne *76, 117*
   interest in Sheila Jones' story *xvi-xvii*,
      153-5
   tribute to Sheila (1999) 83-4
   recollections of Aston (1968) 62
Green, Stuart 154
Greulich, W. 100, *101*
Griffiths, Pam 86
Gulliford, R. 55
Guthrie, Robert 93

Index

Hickmans, Evelyn
   chromatography work 30-3, 118, 135
   dietary work 38, 40-4, 46, 48, 86
   personal notes 132-135
   professional life 12, 13, 14-15, 28-30, 54, 97, 135, 148-9
      commemorative plaque *102*
   receives John Scott Award 98-102
      ceremony photographs 99, *101*
      letters concerning scientific meeting 141-5
      letters of congratulation 138-40
      recollections of Mary Jones 64, 132
      recollections of Sheila 24, 26, 46
      Tom Day on 29
Highcroft Hospital 64-5, 129-30
Hubble, D. 100
Hudson, F.P. 92, 106
Hughes, Patricia 29

inherited metabolic disorders (IMD) 21-2, 80-81, 92, 153
International Society for Neonatal Screening (ISNS) 40, 95
Ireland, Joe 106

Jervis, George 21, 23, 150
John Scott Award (1962) 98-102
   and 25th Anniversary Meeting (1987) 103
   attendees at Scientific Meeting 146
   Birmingham Children's Hospital team awarded 97
      letters received 136-45
      presentation ceremony and speeches 99-102
   notable award winners 98
Jones, Edgar James 4
Jones, Liam 74, 115, *116, 117*
   birth 65, 111
   and Sheila 71, *72, 73*

Jones, Mary (Sheila's mother)
   childhood and arrival in Birmingham 1-4
   marriage 4-6
   gives birth to Sheila 8-9
   single motherhood 6-10, 111-17
   and Sheila's treatment 24, 42-9
      insists on treatment 35-8, 113
      phenylalanine challenge 49-50
      signs of stress 58, 60
   moves family to Aston (1956) 60, 61-4
   mental breakdown 64-5, 100-1
   gives up struggle of Sheila's care 68-70
   visits Sheila at Chelmsley Hospital 71, 75, 114-15
   successfully applies for home visit 71-3
   moves family to Perry Common 74
   death and legacy 75, 118-21
   photographs *xx, 73, 74*
Jones, Philip 65, 72-4, 116, 117
   birth 58, 111
   care in children's homes 65, 115
   with Sheila 72-3
Jones, Sheila
   birth and early behaviour 8-10
      physical characteristics 26
   first admission to BCH (1951) 25-6
   diagnosis from BCH 24-7
      confirmation of PKU 35-8
      diagnostic biochemical results 35, *36, 37*
      gene mutations 109
      question of treatment 38
   second admission to BCH (1951) 42
   BCH treatment (1951-1955) 39-54
      diet preparation 39-54
      phenylalanine free diet, effects of 42-3
      phenylalanine reduced diet 43-4
      diet at home 44-7, 112

weekly visits to BCH 46, 55-6
taking special mixture 46-7
improvement detected 47-8
deterioration as phenylalanine
    reintroduced 49-50
phenylalanine challenge repeated
    51-4
deteriorating dietary control 58-60
home life 112-13
development testing (1952-1955)
    44, 56-9
findings, biochemistry and weight
    charts 53, 59
end of BCH follow up and diet
    59-60
goes to Chelmsley Hospital (1959) 64
admission notes 69-70
first two years 70-1
visit home (1963) 71-3
behaviour (1970s) 73-4
life after mother's death 75-9
character 76, 83
lost in system and re-diagnosis
    (1987) 79-81
develops other medical problems 81
death and tribute to life 83-5
legacy 120-1
Anne Green's interest in *xvi-xvii*,
    153-5
brothers' thoughts on 111-17
Horst Bickle's notes on 135
photographs *viii, 57, 81*
    BCH film *51, 52, 57,* 105
    with brothers Philip and Liam *72*
Jones, Terry, 116, 117
birth 4, 111
care in children's homes 65
family recollections 6, 8, 26, 37-8, 44,
    46, 47, 58, 64-5, 70, 75
early home life 111-17
moving to Aston 63, 114

Jones, Trevor 116, 117
birth 6, 64, 111
family recollections 8, 9-10, 26, 37-8,
    44, 47, 58, 61, 64-5, 68, 70
early home life 111-17
moving to Aston 63, 114
care in children's homes 65
wedding 74
photographs *73, 74, 76, 116, 117*

Kings Norton, Birmingham 4-6
Komrower, George 106

Ladywood Site 11, *12*, 102, 126
Little Bromwich Hospital 55-6, 60, 69
Lordswood Maternity Hospital 8-9
Lunacy Act (1890) 127

MacDonald, Anita 107-8
Marston Green Cottage Homes 66, 129
Mead Johnson 87
Medical Faculty, University of
    Birmingham 99
Medical Research Council 92
Mental Deficiency Act (1913) 66-7, 127, 129
Mental Health Act (1959) 129-30
Mental Health Services 69-70, 79, 127
    Brooklands Hospital 81-3
    Chelmsley Hospital 66-85
    history and changing attitudes 127-30
    testing of females for PKU (1980s) 80
    BCH's assessments of Sheila 56-8
        conclusions about treatment 52-4
        Horst Bickle's notes on 135
    dietary treatment
        importance of continued 119-20
        importance of early 89-90
    early ferric chloride testing 21
        extended to PKU 22-3
        of Sheila 24
Griffiths scale 58

Index

inherited metabolic disorders 21-2, 80-81, 92, 153
   genetic studies 109, 110
   patient care, history 22, 127-30
   phenylpyruvic acid (PPA) 21-2
Merck, Sharp and Dohm 87
methylmalonic acid (MMA) 153

National Health Service (NHS) 13, 120-1, 126, 128
National Society for PKU 95
newborn screening 91-5, 106-7, 121

Oliver, Brian 75
Orthopaedic Hospital 125

Palynziq 109-10
Parsons, Leonard Gregory 12-13, 14, 15, 17, 118, 147-9
Penrose, Lionel 20, 21, 22, 39
Petreus, Laura, and family *104*
Phenistix testing 91-2, 95, 131-2
phenylalanine
   adverse effects on foetus 80
   blood-based screening method 92-6
      challenges 96
   growth, dietary and biochemical control 95-6
   method of removal from natural protein 39-40
      commercial production 86-8
   non PKU individuals 52
   phenylalanine ammonium lyase (PAL) 109-10
   Sheila's PKU diagnosis 35-8
      phenylalanine free and restricted diet *53*
   showing defect in PKU 23, 35, 36
   tetrahydrobiopterin 109
   see also ferric chloride testing and Phenylketonuria (PKU)

Phenylketonuria (PKU)
   awareness of in care facilities 69-70, 79, 100
   characteristic clinical picture of 22
   description of 12 patients at BCH 131
   commercial protein substitutes development 86-8, 107
   advances 88-9
   diagnoses, West Midlands and UK (2018/9) 106
   discovery of 20-2, 150
   early years, history 22-3
   and infant care 96
   enzyme phenylalanine hydroxylase (PAH) 23
   modern treatments 107-10
   and new questions 110
   molecular basis 109
   national register (1963) 92
   National Society for PKU 95
   pregnancy and PKU 80
   screening nationwide
      and dietary treatment 79-80
      newborn screening 91-5, 106-7, 121
   Phenistix testing 91-2, 95, 131-2
   Sheila Jones' case *see* Jones, Sheila
   tyrosine deficiency 23, 35, 38, 41, 43, 48, 134
   see also phenylalanine
phenylpyruvic acid (PPA) 21-2, 30, 35, 43-4, 96
Pollitt, Rodney 153
pregnancy and PKU 80
psychiatric services 128-30

Quastel, J.H. 21, 30
Queen Elizabeth Hospital 126
Queen's Hospital 125

Raine, Noel 93, 106, 107, 135, 153-4
Roy, Ashok 76, 79, 106
Rudd, Brian 29, 33, 34, 43, *103*

Scientific Hospital Supplies (SHS) Ltd 87-8
Scott, John 97
'Scriver' technique *94*, 95
screening nationwide
    and dietary treatment 79-80
    newborn screening 91-5, 106-7, 121
    pregnancy and PKU 80
Selly Oak, Birmingham 2-4
Sheila Jones Award 95, 104-5
Shenley Cottage Homes 65
Smellie, James Maclure 13, 16-7, 25, 55
Smith, Isabel 92
social care services 64, 68, 71, 113
Society for the Study of Inborn Errors of Metabolism (SSIEM) 92
Squire, John 68, *90*, 110-11, 135

St Chads maternity unit 65
Steelhouse Lane site 62, 102, 117

Tonks, Eva 29
tyrosine deficiency *23*, 35, 38, 41, 43, 48, 134

United Birmingham Hospitals Group 13, 140
University of Birmingham and John Scott Award 99-100, 138, 147

Whitehouse, Anne 30, 34
Women's Hospital 125
Women's Royal Voluntary Service (WRVS) 76-7
Wolff, Otto 55
Woolf, Louis 23, 40, 54, 87, 89, 91-2, 106, 118

Youth Training Scheme (YTS) 76